BUDGET
BYTES

BUDGET BYTES

Over **100** Easy, Delicious Recipes
to Slash Your Grocery Bill
– – – – – in Half – – – –

Beth Moncel

AVERY
a member of Penguin Group (USA)
New York

AVERY

Published by the Penguin Group
Penguin Group (USA) LLC
375 Hudson Street
New York, New York 10014

USA · Canada · UK · Ireland · Australia
New Zealand · India · South Africa · China

penguin.com
A Penguin Random House Company

Most Avery books are available at special quantity discounts for bulk purchase for sales promotions, premiums,
fund-raising, and educational needs. Special books or book excerpts also can be created to fit specific needs.
For details, write: Special.Markets@us.penguingroup.com.

Library of Congress Cataloging-in-Publication Data

Moncel, Beth.
Budget bytes : over 100 easy, delicious recipes to slash your grocery bill in half / Beth Moncel.
p.   cm.
ISBN 978-1-58333-530-7 (pbk.)
1. Low budget cooking.   I. Title.
TX714.M658   2014   2013037136
641.5'52—dc23

Printed in the United States of America
3   5   7   9   10   8   6   4

Book design by Meighan Cavanaugh

To all of my readers, who have made my blogging adventure
one of the most valuable and rewarding experiences of my life.
This wouldn't have happened without you.

To my parents, who always made the most of what they had,
even when it wasn't a lot. You were an excellent example.

CONTENTS

- - - - - - - - - -

Introduction   *1*

One
KITCHEN BASICS   *7*

Two
BREAKFAST   *17*

Three
BREADS   *37*

Four
DRESSINGS, DIPS & SAUCES   *61*

Five
SALADS   *79*

Six

PASTA *99*

Seven

SOUPS *119*

Eight

MEAT, POULTRY & SEAFOOD *141*

Nine

RICE, BEANS & LENTILS *179*

Ten

VEGETABLES *197*

Eleven

DESSERTS *215*

Appendix A: Sample Menus *231*

Appendix B: Vegetarian & Vegan Recipes *235*

Appendix C: Volume Conversions *238*

Acknowledgments *239*

Index *240*

INTRODUCTION

-- -- -- -- -- -- -- -- -- -- -- --

I'm not cheap. I like quality things, especially when it comes to food. I also like to pay all of my bills on time without having an anxiety attack the day before payday. The tough part is figuring out how to have both. Having more while cutting back may sound like an oxymoron, but I think I've figured out how to do just that.

In 2009, like many people during the recent recession, I found myself working for low wages and barely making ends meet. I was stuck in a run-down apartment that was smelly, old, and literally falling apart at the seams. I'd always planned on it being a temporary living situation, but when the neighbors' dog caused a building-wide flea infestation, I knew I had to get out, *fast*.

But despite desperately saving my pennies to make the move, student loans were eating me alive, and every time I managed to get a little bit ahead, an unavoidable car repair or medical bill would bring me right back down to zero—or sometimes below. Even everyday items like toothpaste and toilet paper were major expenses that had to be carefully managed to keep my delicate "house of cards" budget from tumbling to the ground.

We've all been there. Household budgets are complex and when unexpected expenses arise, there's a desperate scramble to figure out which necessities can be trimmed. It's not easy, and it definitely isn't fun.

Food is one of the largest daily expenses, but many people feel helpless to cut back on their food budget because of their lack of kitchen skills or the assumption that cooking at home takes too much time or money. So, it's all well-intentioned peanut butter and jelly sandwiches and ramen noodles—at least, until that first real pang of hunger hits. Then it's speed dial for takeout. After all, you've *got* to eat, right?

At that point, my food budget was already pretty meager. A self-proclaimed "Budget Queen," I had just earned a degree in nutritional science for which I'd spent considerable time learning how to create healthy meals on low-income budgets. I dutifully employed the basics, like brown-bagging my lunch, avoiding convenience foods, and cooking meals at home, but it just wasn't enough. Not only was I bored with the food that I ate, but somehow I always seemed to spend more money and waste more food than I meant to or could afford. Certain that I could do more to ease my money problems, I decided to buckle down and crunch the actual numbers . . . like down to the *penny*.

I had taken many foodservice management courses and, while I didn't particularly enjoy them at the time, the lessons suddenly flashed through my mind. I thought about how commercial kitchens managed expenses by planning menus, calculating recipe costs, and *always* repurposing leftovers. *Maybe I could do the same thing in* my *kitchen,* I thought. I knew it was going to take some effort and serious dedication, but hey, I love a good challenge and I desperately needed to save some money! I can't lie—the data geek in me was a little giddy with excitement about the project. So, I started planning, cooking, and calculating.

I initially started with the goal of eating on less than six dollars per day, using Excel to track the cost of every single thing that went in my mouth. It was pure nerdy fun and I was totally into it. The calculations were extremely insightful from the start. I quickly learned which ingredients burned through my food budget and which helped stretch it. Putting my newfound knowledge to work, I was soon cooking twice as much food for half the cost.

At work, my delicious home-cooked lunches started to make my coworkers jealous. While they ate soggy submarine sandwiches, I indulged in stir-fried ginger beef and fragrant jasmine rice. The *ooohs* and *ahhs* that erupted as I heated my homemade lunches let me know that I was onto something. On one particular occasion I was so excited about my low-cost creation that I posted about it on Facebook. Friends started asking for the recipe and that got me thinking . . .

Should I start a blog?

Honestly, I barely knew what a blog was, but I *did* know that the economy had just tanked and I wasn't the only one who might need low-cost recipes. I also knew that the art of cooking had nearly been lost on my generation. When manufacturers start selling microwavable cups of macaroni and cheese because boiling water is too complicated, you know that there is a need for basic cooking instruction. Maybe I could help, by posting my simple, inexpensive recipes and step-by-step instructions. I decided to go for it. And thus, *Budget Bytes* was born.

I was lucky. I grew up in a packed household of seven, where cooking was an everyday event. Cooking for a large family on a tight budget wasn't an easy task, but my mother turned it into something fun and creative. I learned the basics at a very early age and never saw cooking as a grueling task. Instead, it was a science experiment, an art project, or, at the very least, quality time with my mom.

When I started *Budget Bytes*, I wanted people to know that cooking wasn't the laborious chore that it is often made out to be. It can be an enjoyable and rewarding process—and it usually ends with something delicious! I hoped that by giving first-time cooks a little encouragement and guidance, I could help them get over that first hurdle to home cooking.

As it turned out, I severely underestimated the number of people who were in need of easy, delicious, and inexpensive recipes. Just a few short months after I started the blog, comments began to pour in. I got e-mails from all sorts of people who were, like me, struggling to make ends meet, but not willing to sacrifice good food or their whole paycheck to get it. College students, recent graduates, single parents, bachelors, military families, people struggling with medical conditions, and more were all looking for great food on a dime. With every e-mail, every comment, every "thank you" from a reader, I was motivated to create more. The more I created, the more I learned, and the more fun I had sharing what I learned.

For the first time in my life, I loved what I was doing with every ounce of my being. Readers told me they had slashed their grocery bills in half, that they felt more self-sufficient, and that they were now able to spend more quality time with their loved ones.

And my life was changing for the better as well. With the money I saved on my grocery bill, I was able to go back to school, begin a new career, and get out of that horrible little apartment that once served as my motivation. That little project that I had once started to try to make ends meet had blossomed into one of the most rewarding experiences in my life.

Although my budget today is not nearly as tight as it once was, I continue to live and eat by my Budget Byting philosophy and share my experiences with anyone who is interested. *Budget Bytes* continues to grow every day as people around the world decide to take control of their finances and their dinner tables and discover the joys of cooking.

The moral of my story? You don't have to go to cooking school, own fancy kitchen equipment, or spend all day in the kitchen just to make delicious meals at home. I learned how to do it, thousands of my readers have learned how to do it, and you can, too. All it takes is a little practice, dedication, and the confidence to try new things. I've created this book to show people that cooking can be fun, can save you money, and will leave you with both a full belly *and* wallet! This book contains more than one hundred simple, delicious, and incredibly satisfying recipes, and will help you master the techniques to experiment, be creative, and come up with budget creations of your own.

How to Use This Book

The recipes in this book have been designed using the Budget Byting Principles (page 7) to effectively combine ingredients for maximum flavor and minimum cost. Whether you prefer to eat all organic, shop only at local grocers, or just aim for the cheapest option available, you can use the techniques outlined in this book to get the biggest bang for your buck.

Because costs change over time and vary from region to region, no actual dollar amounts are listed with the recipes. Instead, I've created a budget-byting scale to help you pinpoint recipes that fit your budget needs. Each recipe will be placed into one of three categories: Bread 'n' Butter, Frugal Foodie, or Sensible Splurges.

Bread 'n' Butter recipes are the most budget friendly and usually cost around a dollar or less per serving. These recipes rely on basics like pasta, rice, beans, and other pantry staples to fill your belly on a dime. Don't be fooled, though, every recipe packs a flavor punch and will leave your taste buds satisfied! Bread 'n' Butter recipes are designated with a "$" icon.

Frugal Foodie recipes use a few more exotic or exciting ingredients for when you're feeling experimental or have a few extra dollars on hand. Explore new fruits and vegetables, discover ethnic spices, or include a tender cut of meat or two, all while keeping costs under control. Frugal Foodie recipes are designated with a "$$" icon.

Sensible Splurges are recipes for when you really want to indulge. Maybe it's date night, or you're celebrating a birthday, or having a holiday get-together. When you want something extra special you can turn to these recipes without breaking the bank. Sensible Splurges recipes are designated with a "$$$" icon.

In addition to a price category, I've also included Budget Byte tips for finding the best prices and using alternate ingredients to fit specific diet or budget needs. Most recipes are quite flexible and you can use these tips to inspire your own ingredient swaps and creative alterations.

Recipes that are freezer-friendly will be designated with a "❄". This will help you quickly pinpoint recipes that are prime for stocking your freezer with ready-to-go meals. As you'll see, the freezer is one of your best weapons for saving money in the kitchen.

The first chapter includes basic information for those who are new to the kitchen. The "Budget Byting Principles" will help you learn how to shop, eat, and run your kitchen on a budget. "How to Stock a Kitchen" will help you get started by outlining the basic tools and ingredients needed for a well-outfitted kitchen. "Freezer Tips" describes best practices for using your freezer and will help make sure that all the delicious food you're cooking doesn't go to waste. With the information provided in Chapter One, you'll be well on your way to creating great meals and slashing your bills.

In the Appendix, you'll find a few basic menus created using only the recipes in this book. If you're clueless when it comes to pairing side dishes with entrées, check the Appendix for meal ideas that not only taste delicious together, but use ingredients effectively across recipes.

TIPS FOR NEWBIES

I want to offer a few words of wisdom for those who are just beginning their cooking adventure. It can be intimidating, but if you have courage it can be a fun and rewarding experience. Use these tips to make the road a little less bumpy!

1. Always read through a recipe from start to finish before beginning to cook. It's important to understand the flow of a recipe before you begin, and reading it first will prevent surprises that could ruin the outcome.

2. Always preheat your oven. Many of the reactions that occur during cooking and baking rely on exposure to a sudden burst of hot air that can only be achieved with a properly preheated oven. This one simple task can make or break your recipe.

3. Don't sweat ingredient measures. Some ingredients don't always have a precise measurement given (i.e., "freshly cracked pepper, as needed," "1-inch piece fresh ginger"). When an ingredient doesn't have an exact measurement listed, the ingredient is forgiving and the measurement is flexible. If you add a little more or a little less, your recipe won't suffer.

4. Learn from your failures instead of letting them get in the way of your progress. I constantly make mistakes and owe a lot of my knowledge to seeing the results of those missteps. Don't get discouraged, just try again!

One

KITCHEN BASICS

Budget Byting Principles

Learning how to cook on a budget took some practice, but after four years I've come up with these six basic Budget Byting principles by which I shop, cook, and eat to keep my costs under control. If you're new to cooking or just new to working within a budget, these six tips are the perfect place to start.

1. **Plan Your Meals**—There's no way around it. You *have* to take a few minutes to plan ahead. The good news? It gets faster and easier every time you do it! The first step is to choose a few recipes. Pick your recipes based on ingredients that are on sale, produce that is in season, or items you might have on hand. Next, read through the recipes. Check to see what ingredients you already have and make a list of everything that you don't have. Having your recipes chosen and an ingredient list in hand before you set foot in the store is your most powerful weapon. It will prevent you from wandering aimlessly around the store filling your basket with whatever looks good (we've all done it!). *Always* have a plan of attack before you begin.

2. **Use Ingredients Wisely**—Flavorful ingredients are often the most expensive. Fresh herbs, cheese, nuts, and meat all taste great, but also have a large price tag. Stretch the flavor and your dollars by combining those expensive ingredients with bulkier, inexpensive ingredients like pasta, rice, and beans.

Properly combining expensive and inexpensive ingredients can mean having your cake and eating it, too. It's all about the ratio, which can be tweaked to fit the needs of any budget.

3. **Don't Be Afraid of Leftovers**—In an era when the word "fresh" is overused, we've forgotten how wonderful leftovers can be. Leftovers have definitely fallen out of fashion and most people turn up their noses at the thought of them. But sometimes dishes can actually improve with some time in the refrigerator! The flavors mingle and meld, and create new depth. My definition of a good recipe is one that I enjoy eating just as much or even *more* the next day. Sure, not every recipe a good candidate for leftover superstardom, but writing off leftovers altogether is a big mistake. As long as you store your food properly, you can continue to enjoy delicious meals for days, or even longer when frozen.

4. **The Freezer Is Your Friend**—Believe it or not, freezers are good for more than just holding pints of ice cream and keeping your vodka chilled. I keep my freezer stocked at all times with single-serving portions of meals that I use as "grab 'n' go" lunches or backup dinners when I'm just too tired to cook. The freezer will also allow you to take full advantage of sale prices. Meat is usually one of the most expensive ingredients in a recipe, and saving a few dollars per pound can significantly reduce your cost per serving. So, when you see meat (or other expensive ingredients) on sale, grab it, and use your freezer to "save" that sale price for a rainy day.

5. **Shop Around**—Stepping outside of the grocery store box is not only budget savvy, but can also be quite fun. Explore your area for ethnic grocers, produce markets, or community-supported agriculture (CSAs). These hidden gems offer a wide variety of unusual and exciting ingredients, and often at a much lower price than regular grocery stores. Ethnic markets are a great place to find low-price herbs, spices, sauces, and condiments for which regular grocery stores charge a premium. Produce suppliers, farmer's markets, and CSAs are always stocked with in-season produce, which means better quality and lower

prices. So, explore your area for new retailers. You might be surprised at what you find!

6. **Portion Control**—Eating more than you need means, quite literally, spending more than you need. Watching your portions will help keep your waistline small and your wallet fat. I always portion out my meals into single-serving containers as soon as I'm finished cooking to prevent overserving myself later. Aiming for portions that satisfy rather than stuff can stretch your meals twice as far.

How to Stock Your Kitchen

Starting a kitchen from scratch can be a daunting task, but don't worry—you don't have to buy everything all at once! If you start with simple recipes and expand your repertoire slowly from there, you can build up your pantry of ingredients and kitchen tools over time. When I first started out I bought one or two new spices or a small kitchen tool per week and I soon had a well-outfitted kitchen. Go at your own pace and always work within your means. I managed for nearly ten years without a mixer, food processor, or even a proper set of knives, but still made plenty of good food. The comprehensive list below is something to aim for, not what you *need* before beginning. Start small, don't get overwhelmed, and only buy what you truly need at the moment.

Equipment

People were creating delicious food long before there was electricity or fancy-schmancy kitchen gadgets, and you can, too. Basics items like mixing bowls, spoons, spatulas, pots, and pans really are the most important tools in your kitchen.

Sticking to materials like metal, glass, ceramic, and wood is always the best bet. These materials can stand up to a lot of abuse and will last you a lifetime. Plastics may be inexpensive, but they can melt, break, or stain. Fancy-grip rubber handles are just that—fancy—and usually cost much more than they're worth. Take a hint from professional chefs and use basic, no-frills tools that get the job done.

Basic cooking utensils can be purchased for a fair price in most home supply stores, but there are other options if your budget is really tight. Consider restaurant supply stores, after-market or outlet stores, thrift stores, and dollar stores. All of these options can hide excellent deals on basic kitchenware.

Pots and Pans:
2-quart saucepan
6-quart stockpot
10-inch skillet
12-inch skillet (preferably with lid)

Bakeware:
Rimmed baking sheets (set of three)
8-by-8-inch casserole dish
9-by-11-inch casserole dish
9-inch pie dish
Muffin tin

Tools:
Mixing bowl set (glass or stainless steel)
Measuring cups set (¼, ⅓, ½, and 1 cup)
Liquid measuring cup (2-cup volume)
Measuring spoons
Colander
Cutting board
Chef's knife
Bread knife
Mixing spoons, spatulas, whisks

Cheese grater (small- and large-hole)

Aluminum foil

Parchment paper

Plastic wrap

Zip-top freezer bags (gallon- and quart-size)

Resealable storage containers

Pantry Staples

Pantry staples are the ingredients that I like to have on hand at all times. They get wide use in the kitchen and tend to have a long shelf life. Staying stocked up on staples allows you to whip up a variety of recipes on short notice. Make sure to keep these items away from heat and moisture to preserve flavor and prevent spoilage.

Dry Goods:

Flour (all-purpose, whole wheat)

Sugar (white, brown, and powdered)

Rice (white, brown, and jasmine)

Beans (dry or canned)

Pasta

Salt

Baking powder

Baking soda

Oil (vegetable, olive)

Vinegar (apple cider, rice, balsamic)

Honey

Soy sauce

Basic dried herbs and spices (basil, oregano, thyme, chili powder, cayenne, cinnamon, garlic powder)

Refrigerated Items:

Milk

Eggs

Butter

Plain yogurt

Mayonnaise

Dijon mustard

Grated Parmesan cheese

Chicken soup base (such as Better Than Bouillon brand)

Freezer Tips

Without my freezer, I'd have to buy twice as much food and probably give in to takeout at least once a week. Having a freezer allows me to save extra portions of cooked food, save leftover ingredients, and take advantage of sale prices when they're available. But before you start stashing food away in your freezer, there are a few tips and tricks that everyone should know to preserve the flavor, quality, and safety of their food.

Before You Freeze

Divide—Divide food into usable portions prior to freezing. This way you can thaw only the amount that you need and avoid thaw-refreeze cycles. Repeated thawing and freezing of large portions can expose food to dangerous temperatures and degrade the flavor and texture of the food. Divide cooked meals into single-serving portions and divide ingredients (like chicken breasts or chopped vegetables) into portions that would be used for a whole recipe.

Chill—Always chill food in the refrigerator before transferring it to the freezer. When warm or room-temperature foods are placed directly into the freezer, they take longer to freeze and large ice crystals form. Large ice crystals tend to damage food more, resulting in poor texture after thawing. Food that is refrigerated first freezes quickly, forms small ice crystals, and has fewer texture changes.

Package—Choosing the correct packaging for freezing food is important. The main goal of packing food for the freezer is to reduce exposure to air, which can cause moisture loss or freezer burn. Wrap items tightly in plastic and take advantage of thick, freezer-grade zip-top bags. Reusable plastic food storage containers with tight-fitting lids are also excellent for keeping air out and flavor in.

Label—*Always* label your food with the contents and date before freezing. Time flies, and it's very easy to forget when something went into the freezer. While freezing does extend the life of many foods, spoilage still occurs, just at a slower rate.

Freezing Food

Freezer-Friendly Foods—Almost any food can be frozen, but some maintain flavor and texture better than others. Meat, vegetables, cheeses, non-cream-based sauces, and breads are all very freezer-friendly. Frozen vegetables should only be used in dishes where they will be cooked because the freezing process causes them to become soft upon thawing. Despite the texture change, frozen vegetables maintain all of their nutrients and flavor.

Non-Freezer-Friendly Foods—Some foods do not fare well when frozen because they seep water or change texture upon thawing. Cooked eggs can be frozen but tend to seep a small amount of water or become overcooked upon reheating. Mayonnaise and cream-based sauces break down and separate when frozen. Lettuce, which is very delicate and has a high water content, does not hold up well to freezing. Never freeze canned food because the contents will expand upon freezing and may cause the can to burst.

Freezer Limitations—Every food has a different life span when frozen. Some items, like uncooked meat, can be frozen for up to a year, but will slowly diminish in quality. To avoid overstocking my freezer or unintentionally causing waste, I try to use frozen goods within three months from the date on which they were frozen. Take regular inventory of the items in your freezer, so that you don't end up with mystery items or unintentionally purchase items you already have. For specific time ranges for individual foods, consult www.usda.gov.

Using Frozen Food

Thawing—Thawing frozen foods can present multiple food safety issues. The best method for thawing is to place frozen goods in the refrigerator twelve to twenty-four hours prior to use. This allows the food to stay within safe temperature ranges while thawing. The microwave is a suitable option for vegetables or other non-meat items, but make sure to use the thaw setting to prevent partial cooking. Meat and seafood can be quickly thawed under cool running water. Always make sure the water is cool and flowing to prevent dangerous temperatures (between 40 and 140°F) and standing water, both of which promote bacterial growth.

Refreezing—Food that has been thawed can be refrozen as long as it has not reached temperatures above 40°F. This means foods thawed in the microwave or under running water are generally not safe for refreezing. Keep thawing and refreezing to a minimum as this may cause moisture loss and a degradation in quality.

FREEZES GREAT!

- Bread
- Meat, Fish, Poultry
- Cheese

- Butter
- Non-Dairy Sauces
- Cooked Beans
- Cooked Rice
- Soups & Broths
- Casseroles

FREEZES OKAY

- Hearty Vegetables (potatoes, carrots, onions, celery)
- Fresh Herbs
- Pasta
- Milk
- Cooked Eggs
- Fried Food

FREEZES POORLY

- Cream-Based Sauces
- Items Thickened with Gelatin or Cornstarch
- High-Water-Content Vegetables (lettuce, cucumbers, tomatoes)
- Whipped Egg Whites
- Mayonnaise or Mayonnaise-Based Sauces and Dressings

Two

BREAKFAST

We all know that breakfast is the most important meal of the day, but it can be hard to wake up early just to fix something nutritious. Even *I* find it difficult, despite my undying love for breakfast foods. So, to make things easier on myself I've created a collection of breakfast recipes that can be prepared ahead of time and then quickly reheated each morning. I've also included a few specialty items for those lazy weekend mornings when you have time to prepare a little something extra special!

Banana Bread Baked Oatmeal   *18*

Autumn Delight Baked
Oatmeal   *20*

Breakfast Parfaits   *22*

Cranberry-Almond Granola   *24*

Italian Baked Eggs   *26*

Ham & Swiss Crustless Quiche   *27*

Huevos Rancheros Bowls   *29*

Avocado-Egg Toast   *30*

Banana-Nut Muffins   *31*

Iced Orange-Cranberry Scones   *33*

Apple-Cinnamon French Toast
Casserole   *35*

Banana Bread Baked Oatmeal

Serves 6

Baked oatmeal has become a staple in my house. It only takes a few minutes to whip up on Sunday night and then I have a quick microwavable breakfast each morning for the rest of the week. The oats are baked in a lightly sweetened, custardlike mixture that creates a soft, creamy, and totally comforting breakfast treat that will help ease you into the day. It may taste totally indulgent, but it has all the goodness of whole oats!

INGREDIENTS

- 1½ cups mashed bananas (from 3 to 4 medium bananas)
- ⅓ cup packed brown sugar
- 2 large eggs
- ½ teaspoon salt
- ¼ teaspoon ground cinnamon
- ⅛ teaspoon ground nutmeg
- ½ teaspoon vanilla extract
- 1 teaspoon baking powder
- 1½ cups milk
- 2½ cups old-fashioned rolled oats
- ½ cup chopped walnuts

INSTRUCTIONS

Preheat the oven to 375°F. Coat an 8-by-8-inch casserole dish with nonstick cooking spray.

In a large bowl, combine the bananas, brown sugar, eggs, salt, cinnamon, nutmeg, vanilla, and baking powder. Whisk until smooth. Add the milk and whisk again until smooth.

Stir the oats into the banana mixture. Pour the mixture into the prepared casserole dish.

Bake the oatmeal for 45 minutes, or until the top is golden brown and no longer sticky in the center.

Divide the oatmeal into 6 portions and refrigerate or freeze in resealable containers until ready to eat. To reheat, microwave until warmed through.

BUDGET BYTE Purchasing oats from bulk bins not only saves money, but also reduces packaging.

 Chef's Tip: Make sure to buy old-fashioned rolled oats rather than quick-cooking oats. Quick-cooking oats are small and lack the texture needed to stand up to the other ingredients in the recipe.

Chef's Tip: Make sure the bananas are extra ripe. If they still have a touch of green, they won't mash easily, may taste slightly bitter, and won't add enough moisture to the batter.

Autumn Delight Baked Oatmeal $$

Serves 8

This is the Cadillac of baked oatmeal recipes. It combines all of my favorite fall flavors—pumpkin, apple, cranberries, and walnuts—for an incredible amount of flavor and texture. This oatmeal is naturally sweet, super-filling, has tons of fiber, and has all the flavor and aroma of a cozy autumn morning. When you want to treat yourself to something extra-special without breaking your diet, this oatmeal is the ticket.

INGREDIENTS

1 (15-ounce) can pumpkin puree (see Chef's Tip, at right)

2 large eggs

⅓ cup brown sugar

½ teaspoon salt

1 tablespoon ground cinnamon

¼ teaspoon ground cloves

1 teaspoon baking powder

1½ cups milk

1 medium apple, cored and chopped

½ cup chopped walnuts

¼ cup dried cranberries

2½ cups old-fashioned rolled oats

INSTRUCTIONS

Preheat the oven to 375°F. Coat an 8-by-8-inch casserole dish with nonstick cooking spray.

In a large bowl, combine the pumpkin puree, eggs, brown sugar, salt, cinnamon, cloves, and baking powder and whisk until smooth. Add the milk and whisk again until smooth.

Stir the apple, walnuts, cranberries, and oats into the pumpkin mixture. Pour the mixture into the prepared casserole dish.

Bake the oatmeal for 45 minutes, or until the top is slightly golden brown and no longer sticky in the center.

Divide the oatmeal into 8 portions and refrigerate or freeze until ready to eat. To reheat, microwave until warmed through.

Chef's Tip: Pumpkin puree is sometimes labeled "Solid Pack Pumpkin" and should not be confused with "Pumpkin Pie Filling," which is preseasoned and sweetened.

Breakfast Parfaits $

Makes 5

Hot oatmeal is fantastic, but in the dead of summer, a cold breakfast is more appealing. I like to prepare four or five of these on Sunday night and then have breakfast ready and waiting for me in the fridge every morning. As these parfaits refrigerate, the oats absorb moisture from the yogurt and fruit, giving them a unique, chewy texture. In turn, the yogurt thickens up to a creamy Greek yogurt–like consistency. You can customize these parfaits to include just about any fruit or nut you like, but the combination of blueberry, pineapple, almond, and flaxseed is my favorite!

INGREDIENTS

2½ cups plain or vanilla yogurt

1⅔ cups old-fashioned rolled oats

1¼ teaspoons ground cinnamon

5 tablespoons ground flaxseed

5 tablespoons sliced almonds

1¼ cups frozen blueberries

1 (15-ounce) can pineapple chunks in juice, drained, juice reserved (see Budget Byte, at right)

INSTRUCTIONS

In each of 5 (12-ounce) lidded Mason jars, layer ½ cup yogurt, ⅓ cup oats, ¼ teaspoon cinnamon, 1 tablespoon flaxseed, and 1 tablespoon sliced almonds.

Add ¼ cup of the blueberries to each jar. Divide the pineapple chunks evenly among the jars.

Refrigerate the jars overnight before serving to allow the oats to absorb moisture and soften. Stir just before eating.

 Chef's Tip: Mason jars are perfect for these parfaits because they're portable and reusable, and the chilled glass will keep the parfait cold as you eat.

BUDGET BYTE The leftover pineapple juice is excellent for making smoothies. Store the juice in an airtight container in the refrigerator for up to 1 week or in the freezer for up to 3 months.

Cranberry-Almond Granola $

Serves 8   I'm always surprised at how expensive prepackaged granola is. Sure, it has some pricier ingredients, like dried fruit and nuts, but the bulk of granola is very inexpensive ingredients like oats, sugar, and oil. Making granola at home is easy and customizable, and makes your house smell delicious. Just be careful—with all of this yummy, inexpensive granola around, you might find yourself snacking on it nonstop!

INGREDIENTS

4 cups old-fashioned rolled oats

⅓ cup dried cranberries

⅓ cup sliced almonds

⅓ cup ground flaxseed

¼ cup vegetable oil

¼ cup honey

½ cup brown sugar

½ teaspoon almond extract

½ teaspoon vanilla extract

¼ teaspoon salt

INSTRUCTIONS

Preheat the oven to 325°F. Line a rimmed baking sheet with parchment paper.

In a large bowl, stir together the oats, cranberries, almonds, and flaxseed until combined.

In a small saucepan, combine the vegetable oil, honey, brown sugar, almond extract, vanilla, and salt with ¼ cup of water and cook over medium heat, stirring, until liquid and combined. The sugar may not completely dissolve, but the mixture should be heated to the point where it is easily pourable.

Pour the sugar mixture into the oat mixture and stir until evenly coated. Pour the granola onto the lined baking sheet and spread it into an even layer.

Bake the granola for 40 minutes. Use the back of a spatula to press the granola down into a compact layer; this will help the granola form clumps as it cools. Allow the granola to cool completely, then break it into chunks. Store the granola in an airtight container at room temperature.

 BUDGET BYTE Bulk bins are a great place to find a variety of granola add-ins for low prices.

Italian Baked Eggs $

Serves 4

This is a really simple way to turn a humble egg-and-toast breakfast into something extraordinary. Plus, it's a great way to use up the leftover pasta sauce that always seems to linger in the back of the refrigerator. You can make the recipe for four, as listed, or easily scale it up or down to feed any number of people. If you don't have ramekins, an oven-safe mug will also do the job.

INGREDIENTS

1 teaspoon salted butter

1 cup marinara sauce

¼ cup grated Parmesan

4 large eggs

Salt

Ground black pepper

Fresh parsley, for garnish (optional)

Toast, for serving

INSTRUCTIONS

Preheat the oven to 375°F. Butter 4 (6-ounce) ramekins (use your fingers or a small piece of plastic wrap to help you smear the butter over the inside surface of the ramekin).

Place 3 tablespoons of the marinara sauce in the bottom of each ramekin, followed by 1 tablespoon of the Parmesan. Crack 1 egg into each ramekin and season each egg with salt and pepper to taste. Top each egg with 1 tablespoon of the remaining marinara sauce.

Place the ramekins into a baking dish (for easy transport in and out of the oven) and bake for 18 to 20 minutes, or until the egg yolk is lightly set. Garnish with fresh parsley, if desired. Serve with toast for dipping.

Ham & Swiss Crustless Quiche $$

Serves 6

I love savory breakfasts. They're ultra-satisfying and usually high in protein, which keeps me full for hours. The high-fat-content crust on quiche can make me feel guilty, so one day I just skipped the crust, and I've never looked back! Similar to a frittata, but with a more custardlike filling, this crustless quiche has both protein and vegetables to keep you fueled all morning.

INGREDIENTS

1 tablespoon vegetable oil

1 small yellow onion, diced

½ pound smoked deli ham, sliced into 1-inch strips

8 ounces frozen chopped spinach, thawed

1 cup shredded Swiss cheese

4 large eggs

¾ cup milk

¼ cup grated Parmesan

Pinch of freshly cracked black pepper

1 small tomato, sliced

INSTRUCTIONS

Preheat the oven to 350°F. Coat a 9-inch pie dish with nonstick cooking spray and set the pie dish on a rimmed baking sheet.

In a medium skillet, heat the vegetable oil over medium heat. Add the onion and sauté for about 5 minutes, until soft and translucent. Add the ham and sauté for 5 minutes more. Spread the cooked onions and ham in an even layer over the bottom of the prepared pie dish.

Place the thawed spinach in a colander and squeeze out as much moisture as possible. Lay the spinach in an even layer over the onions and ham in the pie dish. Sprinkle half of the Swiss cheese over the spinach.

In a medium bowl, whisk together the eggs, milk, Parmesan, and pepper. Pour the egg mixture into the pie dish. Arrange the tomato slices over the top of the unbaked quiche. Sprinkle the remaining Swiss cheese over the tomatoes.

Bake for 40 minutes, or until the center has puffed and the outer edges are slightly golden brown.

Allow the quiche to rest for 5 minutes before slicing and serving. Uneaten portions can be refrigerated in resealable containers for up to 5 days.

 Chef's Tip: Deli meat contains a surprising amount of moisture, so it's important to sauté the ham before adding it to the quiche to prevent a soggy quiche bottom.

Huevos Rancheros Bowls $$

Serves 4

I'm obsessed with tacos. Huevos rancheros are a lot like tacos, but topped with an egg, which makes me love them even more! Unfortunately, I find huevos rancheros slightly difficult to eat. I can never get everything I want into one bite, so I created an easier-to-eat "bowl" version of the dish by replacing the crispy tortilla with corn grits. It's definitely a winner.

INGREDIENTS

¾ cup dry yellow grits

¼ teaspoon salt

½ cup shredded cheddar

4 large eggs

1 cup black beans

1 cup salsa

1 ripe medium avocado, diced

INSTRUCTIONS

In a medium saucepan, bring 3 cups of water to a boil over high heat. Stir in the grits and salt. Reduce the heat to low, cover the pan, and simmer for 5 to 7 minutes, or until the grits have thickened. Remove the pan from the heat and stir in the cheddar.

While the grits are cooking, fry the eggs.

Place ¾ cup of the grits in each of 4 bowls, then top each with a fried egg, ¼ cup of the black beans, ¼ cup of the salsa, and one-quarter of the diced avocado.

 Chef's Tip: To prepare this ahead of time, build the Huevos Rancheros bowls, minus the egg, in individual resealable containers, which can then be stored in the refrigerator. Each morning, simply reheat a container in the microwave and add a freshly fried egg.

Avocado-Egg Toast $

I'm addicted to egg-and-cheese breakfast sandwiches, but they're not the healthiest option around. When I discovered that avocado provides the same delicious creamy texture as cheese but with much healthier fats, I fell in *love*. Avocado-Egg Toast became my favorite summertime breakfast quick fix. Sometimes I serve this over a slice of whole-wheat toast, other times I stuff it all inside a multigrain pita. Sometimes with hot sauce, sometimes without. The choice is yours.

INGREDIENTS

1 large egg

Pinch of salt

Pinch of ground black pepper

¼ ripe medium avocado

1 slice hearty whole-wheat toast or
    pita pocket

Hot sauce (sriracha, Tabasco, or your
    favorite brand; optional)

INSTRUCTIONS

Fry the egg and season it with the salt and pepper.

Smash the avocado and spread it over the toast. Sprinkle it with a touch of hot sauce and top it with the fried egg.

 Chef's Tip: After you've cut the portion of avocado you need for this recipe, sprinkle lemon juice over the cut surface of the remaining avocado to keep it from browning. Store the cut avocado in a resealable container in the refrigerator for up to 5 days.

Banana-Nut Muffins

$

Everyone needs a good, basic banana muffin recipe. Not only are they a classic comfort food, but we all have overripe bananas begging to be saved from the Dumpster from time to time. Make a batch of these muffins and store them in the freezer. A quick 30 seconds in the microwave takes them from frozen to warm and ready to eat when you're sleepy and bleary-eyed in the morning.

Makes 12

INGREDIENTS

1½ cups all-purpose flour

½ cup whole-wheat flour

2 teaspoons baking powder

½ teaspoon salt

1½ cups mashed bananas (from 3 to 4 ripe medium bananas; see Chef's Tip, page 32)

2 tablespoons vegetable oil

2 large eggs

½ cup sugar

½ cup milk

½ teaspoon vanilla extract

½ teaspoon ground cinnamon

⅛ teaspoon ground nutmeg

½ cup walnuts, chopped

INSTRUCTIONS

Preheat the oven to 350°F. Line a 12-cup muffin tin with paper liners or coat each well with nonstick cooking spray.

In a large bowl, combine the all-purpose flour, whole-wheat flour, baking powder, and salt and stir until evenly combined.

In a separate large bowl, combine the bananas, vegetable oil, eggs, sugar, milk, vanilla, cinnamon, and nutmeg and whisk until smooth. Stir in the chopped walnuts.

Combine the banana mixture with the flour mixture and stir just until everything has been moistened. Do not overmix; this can cause the finished muffin to have a rubbery texture.

Divide the batter evenly among the wells of the muffin tin. Bake for 27 to 30 minutes, or until the muffins are puffed up and golden brown on top. Set the muffin tin on a wire rack and allow to cool before eating.

 Chef's Tip: Make sure the bananas are extra ripe. If they still have a touch of green, they won't mash easily, may taste slightly bitter, and won't add enough moisture to the batter.

Iced Orange-Cranberry Scones

Once you discover how incredibly fast and easy scones are to make, you'll never pay $2.50 *Makes 8* for one at your local coffee shop again. These scones bake up light and crumbly with the fragrant scent of orange and the occasional sweet-tart bite of a dried cranberry. These fancy-pants pastries will take your morning coffee or afternoon tea up a notch *without* breaking the bank.

INGREDIENTS

2 cups all-purpose flour, plus more for dusting

2 tablespoons granulated sugar

2 teaspoons baking powder

½ teaspoon salt

1 medium orange

5 tablespoons salted butter, cold

⅓ cup dried cranberries

3 tablespoons milk

2 large eggs

1 cup powdered sugar

INSTRUCTIONS

Preheat the oven to 450°F. Line a baking sheet with parchment paper.

In a large bowl, combine the flour, granulated sugar, baking powder, and salt. Using a Microplane or a small-holed cheese grater, scrape off the thin, orange layer of zest from the orange (do not grate down to the white pith). Stir the orange zest into the flour mixture. Reserve the orange.

Cut the butter into chunks and add it to the flour mixture. Use your hands to work the butter into the flour until it resembles coarse sand. Stir in the cranberries.

In a small bowl, whisk together the milk and eggs. Pour the milk and eggs into the flour mixture. Stir until everything comes together into a lump of dough.

Dust a clean work surface with flour. Turn the dough out onto the floured work surface and shape it into a circle, about 8 inches in diameter and 1 inch thick. Cut the circle evenly into 8 wedges and transfer them to the lined baking sheet, arranging them a couple inches apart from one another.

Bake for 13 to 15 minutes, or until lightly golden brown on top.

Remove from the oven and allow the scones to cool completely.

Cut the reserved orange in half and squeeze the juice from one half into a small bowl. In a separate small bowl, combine the powdered sugar and 1 tablespoon of the orange juice and stir until smooth. (Reserve the remaining orange juice for another use.) Once the scones have cooked to room temperature, drizzle the icing over the top.

 Chef's Tip: Make sure the butter is cold so that it does not melt into the flour. Small, pea-size chunks of butter give the scone a more flaky, crumbly texture.

 Chef's Tip: In place of the icing, coarse sugar can be sprinkled over the top of each scone before baking.

Apple-Cinnamon French Toast Casserole $

This may not be an everyday breakfast item, but for special occasions like birthdays, holidays, or a smorgasbord brunch, this French toast casserole is perfect. It's rich, sweet, and has a wonderfully crunchy streusel topping. Say hello to your new favorite way to eat French toast!

Serves 6

INGREDIENTS

3 large eggs

1½ cups milk

6 tablespoons brown sugar

1 teaspoon vanilla extract

¼ teaspoon salt

½ teaspoon ground cinnamon

12 (1-inch-thick) slices soft French bread (from about ½ large loaf)

1 medium Granny Smith apple, sliced into wedges

¼ cup old-fashioned rolled oats

2 tablespoons salted butter, room temperature

INSTRUCTIONS

Preheat the oven to 350°F. Spray an 8-by-8-inch casserole dish with nonstick cooking spray.

In a medium bowl, whisk together the eggs, milk, 2 tablespoons of the brown sugar, the vanilla, salt, and cinnamon.

Dip each slice of bread into the egg mixture and let it to soak for a second or two on each side. Place the soaked bread slices in two rows of six inside the casserole dish, slightly overlapping them like fallen dominos. Tuck apple wedges between each slice of soaked French bread. Pour any remaining egg mixture over top. If needed, the dish can be covered and refrigerated for up to 12 hours at this point.

Mix the streusel topping just before baking. In a small bowl, combine the rolled oats, the remaining 4 tablespoons brown sugar, and the butter and stir until the mixture has a slightly crumbly texture. Sprinkle the streusel mixture over the top of the casserole.

Bake for 45 minutes, or until the streusel topping is golden brown and crisp. Serve 2 slices of French toast per person.

Three

BREADS

Baking bread is a truly magical experience. The therapeutic act of kneading, watching the bread rise, and the amazing smell that fills your house as it bakes are all experiences that can't be matched. Many people are intimidated by bread, but I've included recipes to match every skill level. If you're new to bread, start by reading through the bread basics and then try your hand at a simple, quick bread recipe like Parmesan-Herb Drop Biscuits (page 43). Once you're ready to experiment with yeast, try out a no-knead yeast bread like my famous No-Knead Focaccia (page 48). Finally, when you've gained some bread-baking confidence, dive in with a classic yeast bread recipe like my Honey-Wheat Sandwich Bread (page 50). You'll be a master breadmaker in no time!

QUICK BREADS

Honey-Wheat Biscuits   *41*

Parmesan-Herb Drop Biscuits   *43*

Jalapeño Cornbread   *45*

Cheddar-Beer Bread   *47*

YEAST BREADS

No-Knead Focaccia   *48*

Honey-Wheat Sandwich Bread   *50*

Soft 'n' Sweet Dinner Rolls   *52*

Multigrain Rolls   *54*

Naan   *56*

Italian Breadsticks   *58*

BREAD BASICS

If you're new to baking bread, take a few minutes to review this basic information. These quick tips and definitions will help demystify the bread-baking process and ease your transition into a master breadmaker! Okay, maybe that's a bit lofty, but it will definitely make the process a little less intimidating. Promise.

Quick Bread, Yeast Bread

Some bread recipes use yeast to make them rise, some don't. Recipes that don't use yeast are generally referred to as quick breads. Biscuits, muffins, cakes, and banana bread all fall into this category. Quick breads rely on steam and gas produced by acid-base reactions to make them light and fluffy. These reactions happen quickly compared to gas production by yeast, hence the name "quick bread." Baking soda or baking powder usually acts as the base in these chemical reactions, and lemon juice, buttermilk, or vinegar usually acts as the acid. Placing a quick-bread batter into a very hot oven also produces a sudden burst of steam that then gets trapped in the bread as the batter sets—hence the importance of preheating the oven!

Rather than quick acid-base reactions, yeast breads rely on gas produced by yeast to make them rise. Yeast produces gas when it digests carbohydrates, but this reaction is slow and can take hours to make a loaf rise. Yeast bread recipes use a thick dough, rather than a batter, which is needed to hold in the gas during the long rising process. A protein called gluten provides strength and structure to yeast bread dough, as well as its characteristically chewy texture. Kneading bread dough forms a strong gluten lattice, which enhances this texture.

All About Yeast

There are several types of yeast on the market, and it's important to be aware of which type you are using. Most yeast used today is dry and sold in either packets or small jars. Both instant and active dry yeast are sold in this form. Although they look exactly alike, they act quite different. Active dry yeast must be dissolved in water and allowed to activate or "proof" for a few minutes before it can be added to a recipe. Instant yeast does not require proofing and can be added to a recipe dry. The recipe method will determine which type of yeast can be used. In recipes that include a proofing step, both active dry and instant yeast will work. Recipes that skip proofing and combine all of the dough ingredients in one step, like bread machine or no-knead recipes, will only work with instant yeast.

Individual packets of yeast are ¼ ounce in weight, or approximately 2¼ teaspoons in volume. One envelope of yeast can be used for any recipe in this book that calls for 2 teaspoons of yeast. Although yeast envelopes are convenient, I like to purchase small, 4-ounce jars of yeast (usually sold right next to the envelopes) because they are more economical. When refrigerated, a jar of yeast will remain viable for about a year, and it allows you to use any amount needed for a recipe.

Yeast Quick List

- **Active Dry Yeast:** Must be activated by dissolving in warm water before adding to a recipe.
- **Instant Yeast:** Can be added to a recipe dry, without dissolving in warm water first. This is the type of yeast most commonly used for "no-knead" bread recipes and in bread machines.
- **Bread Machine Yeast:** This is the same as instant yeast and does not need to be dissolved in warm water before adding to a recipe.
- **Rapid-Rise Yeast:** Another name for instant yeast. This yeast does not need to be dissolved in water before adding to a recipe.
- **Cake or Fresh Yeast:** This type of yeast is highly perishable and generally used only in commercial kitchens. Although it works faster and longer than dry forms of yeast, it must be refrigerated and is hard to find in most grocery stores.

Kneading Dough

Kneading bread dough is like riding a bike. It may seem awkward at first, but once you get the rhythm down, it becomes automatic. Kneading is necessary to achieve the light, fluffy, and slightly chewy texture that is characteristic of great bread. It also helps ensure that all the ingredients are thoroughly mixed. Kneading will allow you to work more flour into the dough once it becomes too thick to stir with a spoon. Bread that is properly kneaded is soft, smooth, and buoyant. When dough is sufficiently kneaded, it should spring back quickly when poked with a finger. A minimum of five minutes of kneading is usually necessary to achieve this texture.

So how do you knead dough? The basic technique, done on a flat, floured surface, involves folding the dough in half, pressing it down and forward, giving it a quarter turn and repeating the process again and again. Flour should be occasionally sprinkled on the work surface to keep the dough from sticking. If too much flour is added, the dough can become dry and stiff, so add flour only when necessary. If you're a visual learner, I highly recommend doing a quick Internet search for videos demonstrating kneading techniques.

Let It Rise

Allowing yeast dough to rise is called "proofing" the dough. Most yeast bread recipes call for allowing the dough to rise twice, doubling in volume each time. The amount of time needed for bread dough to double in size will vary depending on the ambient room temperature and humidity. I find that temperatures above 70°F work best for allowing dough to rise, while temperatures lower than this can dramatically increase the amount of time needed. During the winter months, or if your house is unusually cool, you can proof the bread dough in an oven with the power turned off and a dish of steaming hot water to slightly increase the ambient air temperature.

Baking bread is an art form because it takes practice and intricate knowledge. The more you practice, the easier it will get, and soon you'll walk past those squishy, lackluster loaves in the grocery store without a second glance.

Honey-Wheat Biscuits

$

A basic biscuit recipe should be in every cook's arsenal. They're fast, easy, and an incredible treat on a lazy weekend morning. These tall, fluffy biscuits are moist and sweet, thanks to a touch of honey, and have a little extra flavor, texture, and fiber from the whole-wheat flour. The unbaked biscuits can be frozen and baked as needed straight from the freezer. Just increase the cooking time by 3 to 5 minutes.

Makes 12

INGREDIENTS

1½ cups all-purpose flour, plus more for dusting

1 cup whole-wheat flour

1 tablespoon baking powder

1 teaspoon salt

6 tablespoons salted butter, cold

¼ cup honey

¾ cup milk

INSTRUCTIONS

Preheat the oven to 400°F. Line a baking sheet with parchment paper.

In a large bowl, combine the all-purpose flour, whole-wheat flour, baking powder, and salt and stir until well combined.

Cut the butter into small pieces and add them to the flour mixture. Use your hands to work the butter into the flour until no large chunks remain and the mixture resembles coarse sand.

In a small bowl, whisk together the honey and milk. Pour the honey mixture into the flour mixture and stir until a dough forms and no dry flour remains on the bottom of the bowl.

Lightly dust a clean work surface with flour. Turn the dough out onto the floured surface and use a rolling pin to roll the dough out into a ¼-inch-thick rectangle. Fold it into thirds like a letter, then roll it out into a ¼-inch-thick rectangle a second time. Fold the dough into thirds once again, then roll it out into a ¾-inch-thick rectangle. (This folding process will create flaky layers in the biscuits.)

Cut the dough into 12 squares, or use a biscuit cutter to cut 12 dough circles. Place the biscuits on the lined baking sheet.

Bake for about 12 minutes, or until the biscuits have puffed up and are golden brown on top. Serve warm.

 BUDGET BYTE If 12 biscuits is too many for you to consume, freeze the unbaked biscuits between layers of parchment paper in a gallon-size freezer bag. The frozen biscuits can then be baked one at a time or in whatever quantity is needed, straight from the freezer.

Parmesan-Herb Drop Biscuits

$

These are the best biscuits I've ever had. I just need to let you know that up front. Not only are they the best biscuits I've ever had, but they're also the *easiest* biscuits I've ever *made*. Simply mix the dough, plop it by the spoonful onto the baking sheet, and 18 to 20 minutes later you have a light, fluffy biscuit with BIG flavor. They're so delicious that no one will ever guess how easy they are to make.

Makes 10

INGREDIENTS

2 cups all-purpose flour

¼ cup grated Parmesan

⅛ teaspoon garlic powder

½ teaspoon dried oregano

½ teaspoon dried basil

1 teaspoon sugar

1 tablespoon baking powder

½ teaspoon salt

8 tablespoons salted butter, cold

1 cup milk

INSTRUCTIONS

Preheat the oven to 400°F. Line a baking sheet with parchment paper.

In a large bowl, combine the flour, Parmesan, garlic powder, oregano, basil, sugar, baking powder, and salt and stir until well combined.

Cut the butter into small pieces and add it to the flour mixture. Use your hands to work the butter into the flour mixture until the butter is in very small pieces and the texture resembles coarse sand.

Starting with ¾ cup of the milk, stir in just enough milk to form a thick, pastelike mixture. It should be very wet, sticky, and soft enough to scoop with a spoon.

Scoop ⅓-cup portions of the dough onto the lined baking sheet. You should have enough dough for 10 biscuits.

Bake for 18 to 20 minutes, or until the biscuits have puffed up and are golden brown on top. Serve warm.

BUDGET BYTE This recipe can easily be scaled down if you're cooking for just one, two, or three. Simply divide all the ingredients in half and follow the directions as written.

Chef's Tip: If you don't have the exact mix of herbs I've used here, feel free to experiment with your own combination!

Jalapeño Cornbread

 $ ❄

Serves 9

I used to be a boxed-mix cornbread addict. I loved the stuff. It was easy, cheap, and delicious, or so I thought. Then one day I finally decided to try to make it from scratch. To my surprise, it was every bit as easy as the boxed mix and *so* much better tasting. I like to add fresh jalapeño to my cornbread because it adds a little kick and a wonderfully fresh flavor. You can control the amount of heat in the bread by increasing or decreasing the amount of jalapeño seeds added to the batter. For mild cornbread, remove all the seeds; for spicy bread, leave some of the seeds in.

INGREDIENTS

1 cup yellow cornmeal

1 cup all-purpose flour

¼ cup sugar

1 tablespoon baking powder

½ teaspoon salt

1 large egg

1 cup milk

¼ cup vegetable oil

2 medium jalapeños

INSTRUCTIONS

Preheat the oven to 425°F. Coat an 8-by-8-inch baking dish or 9-inch pie dish with nonstick cooking spray.

In a large bowl, combine the cornmeal, flour, sugar, baking powder, and salt and stir until well combined.

In a small bowl, whisk together the egg, milk, and vegetable oil.

Cut the jalapeños in half and scrape the seeds out with a spoon. Alternatively, leave some seeds in if you want a little heat. Dice the peppers and stir them into the egg mixture.

Pour the egg mixture into the cornmeal mixture and stir just until everything is moistened. Do not overmix. Pour the batter into the prepared pan.

Bake for 25 minutes, or until the bread is slightly browned around the edges and a toothpick inserted in the center comes out clean.

 Chef's Tip: To make corn muffins, divide the batter between 9 wells in a muffin tin and bake for 18 to 20 minutes, or until golden brown.

Cheddar-Beer Bread $$

This is a truly indulgent quick bread. It's rich, slightly sweet, and has that earthy beer flavor, which makes it perfect for sopping up winter soups and stews. You can change the flavor of the bread by using different varieties of beer, but I find that full-bodied wheat lagers provide a nice, deep flavor. Although it mixes up quickly, the bread does need some time in the oven, so start this bread before you begin making dinner and it will be ready when you are.

Serves 8

INGREDIENTS

3 cups all-purpose flour

¼ cup sugar

1 tablespoon baking powder

1 teaspoon salt

1 cup shredded cheddar

12 ounces beer

INSTRUCTIONS

Preheat the oven to 350°F. Coat a loaf pan with nonstick cooking spray.

In a large bowl, combine the flour, sugar, baking powder, and salt and stir until well combined. Add the cheese and stir until incorporated.

Pour the beer into the flour mixture and stir just until everything is moistened. Pour the batter into the prepared pan.

Bake for 50 minutes, or until the top of the bread is golden brown.

 Chef's Tip: For an extra-decadent beer bread, pour a few tablespoons of melted butter over the batter in the pan before baking.

No-Knead Focaccia

Serves 12

This no-knead focaccia is the perfect yeast bread for beginners. Although it takes a little time to work its magic (you'll need to start it the day before), the dough pretty much does all the work itself. Allowing the dough to ferment develops both the flavor and gluten, which gives bread a wonderful flavor and texture. Because the yeast has so much time to work its magic and multiply, only a scant ¼ teaspoon is needed for the entire batch, making this bread even more economical. Focaccia is my favorite bread for sandwiches, but it also makes a hearty accompaniment to soups and stews. You're going to love this easy, flavorful focaccia!

INGREDIENTS

1 cup whole-wheat flour

3 cups all-purpose flour

1½ teaspoons salt

¼ teaspoon instant yeast

2 tablespoons cornmeal

2 tablespoons olive oil

1 tablespoon Italian seasoning blend

INSTRUCTIONS

In a large bowl, combine the whole-wheat flour, all-purpose flour, salt, and yeast and stir until well combined. Starting with 1½ cups, stir in just enough water to form a cohesive ball of dough; you may need up to 2 cups. There should be no dry flour on the bottom of the bowl. It's okay if the dough is slightly wet and sticky.

Cover the bowl loosely with plastic wrap and set aside to rest for 12 to 18 hours at room temperature. The dough will expand and become bubbly as it ferments.

Line a baking sheet with foil, coat the foil with nonstick cooking spray, and then sprinkle it lightly with the cornmeal. Liberally sprinkle flour on top of the dough to keep your hands from sticking and carefully scrape the dough out of the bowl and onto the baking sheet. Stretch and pat the dough out into a rectangle to fit the baking sheet. Stretch it all the way to the edges, if possible.

Drizzle the surface with olive oil and spread it around with your fingers. Sprinkle the Italian seasoning blend over the top. Set the dough aside to rise at room temperature for 1 hour.

Preheat the oven to 425°F.

Use your fingers to press dimples into the surface of the dough. Bake for 20 to 25 minutes, or until the surface is golden brown.

Transfer the focaccia from the baking sheet to a wire rack as it cools to prevent condensation. Allow the focaccia to cool to room temperature before slicing it into 12 squares.

 Chef's Tip: It is important to use instant yeast for this recipe rather than active dry yeast. Unlike active dry yeast, instant yeast does not need to be dissolved in water prior to being added to a recipe.

 Chef's Tip: The flavor of this bread can be customized by topping with any of your favorite ingredients like cheese, dried fruit, or nuts.

Honey-Wheat Sandwich Bread

*Makes
1 loaf*

This is my favorite basic bread recipe. It uses a combination of whole-wheat and all-purpose flours to yield a bread that has plenty of flavor and texture, but is still light and fluffy. The honey provides just a hint of sweetness, but the flavor is neutral enough for everything from a turkey sandwich to toast with jam.

INGREDIENTS

2 teaspoons active dry or
   instant yeast

1¼ cups warm water

2 tablespoons honey

3 tablespoons olive oil

½ tablespoon salt

1½ cups whole-wheat flour

2 to 3 cups all-purpose flour

INSTRUCTIONS

In a small bowl, combine the yeast and warm water. Stir until the yeast has dissolved and then set aside for 5 minutes, or until the mixture becomes thick and frothy on top. Stir in the honey, olive oil, and salt.

Place the whole-wheat flour in a large bowl. Add the yeast mixture and stir until smooth. Begin adding the all-purpose flour, ½ cup at a time, until the dough becomes too thick to stir with a spoon.

Turn the dough out onto a clean work surface. Sprinkle the work surface lightly with flour and knead the dough for 5 minutes, adding small amounts of flour as you go. When the dough is fully kneaded, it should be smooth, no longer sticky, and will bounce back when poked with a finger. Approximately 2½ cups of all-purpose flour should be added to the dough in total, although the exact amount may vary slightly depending on the humidity and moisture level in your flour (you may not use all the flour).

Place the dough back into the mixing bowl, cover it loosely with plastic, and let it rise for 1 hour, or until doubled in volume.

Coat a loaf pan with nonstick cooking spray. Punch down the dough and shape it into a log the same length as your loaf pan. Transfer the dough to the prepared pan and set aside to rise for 1 hour more, or until doubled in volume.

Preheat the oven to 425°F.

Bake the bread for 30 minutes, or until golden brown on top. Remove the pan from the oven and place it on a wire rack. Let cool to room temperature before slicing.

 Chef's Tip: Always allow bread to fully cool before cutting into it to prevent it from collapsing or losing moisture.

 This bread can be frozen for up to 3 months. Thaw it in the refrigerator or at room temperature until soft.

Soft 'n' Sweet Dinner Rolls

$

Makes 12

When I first tested this recipe, I knew I had stumbled upon something really dangerous. These rolls are light, fluffy, just a little bit sweet, and completely addicting. They're perfect slathered with some warm, melty butter, and have comfort written all over them. I knew I had to get them out of the house before I ate the whole batch, so I called up my landlord, who literally *ran* over to get them. I'm pretty sure these rolls won me the "best tenant of the year" award.

INGREDIENTS

2 teaspoons active dry yeast

¾ cup warm water

1 large egg

2 tablespoons salted butter, melted

3 tablespoons sugar

1 teaspoon salt

3 cups all-purpose flour

INSTRUCTIONS

In a small bowl, combine the yeast and water. Stir until the yeast has dissolved and then set aside for 5 minutes, or until the mixture becomes thick and frothy on top. Add the egg, butter, and sugar and whisk until smooth.

In a large bowl, combine the salt and 1 cup of the flour and stir until evenly combined. Pour the yeast mixture into the flour mixture and stir until smooth.

Add the remaining flour, ½ cup at a time, until you can no longer stir the mixture with a spoon. Turn out the dough onto a clean work surface and knead for about 5 minutes, adding more flour as needed to prevent the dough from sticking. When fully kneaded, the dough will be soft, smooth, and not sticky; you may not need to use all of the flour.

Return the kneaded dough to the mixing bowl, cover it loosely with plastic, and let rise for 1 hour, or until doubled in volume.

Line a large baking sheet with parchment paper. Punch down the dough and transfer it to a clean, floured work surface. Divide the dough into 12 pieces and shape each piece into a small ball. Arrange the dough balls on the lined baking sheet. Allow the rolls to rise for 1 hour more, or until doubled in volume.

While the rolls are rising, preheat the oven to 400°F.

Bake for 10 to 12 minutes, or until golden brown on top. Serve warm.

Multigrain Rolls

Makes 12

I love hearty artisan bread, the kind that is chock-full of seeds, grains, and texture. I made these rolls to mimic my favorite grocery store artisan bread, but they're completely customizable. Simply mix up one cup total of your favorite bran, seeds, or nuts and add them into this basic whole-wheat dough for a super-texture-licious roll. Take advantage of bulk bins at the grocery store to get a variety of add-ins for a low price and in the exact amount that you need.

INGREDIENTS

1½ teaspoons instant or active
   dry yeast

1½ cups warm water

1 tablespoon sugar

1 tablespoon olive oil

1 cup whole-wheat flour

¼ cup wheat or oat bran

¼ cup ground flaxseed

¼ cup raw sunflower seeds

¼ cup sesame seeds

1 teaspoon salt

2 to 3 cups all-purpose flour

INSTRUCTIONS

In a small bowl, combine the yeast, warm water, and sugar. Stir to dissolve the yeast and then set aside for 5 minutes, or until the mixture becomes thick and frothy on top. Stir in the olive oil. In a large bowl, combine the whole-wheat flour, bran, flaxseed, sunflower seeds, sesame seeds, and salt and stir until evenly combined. Pour the yeast mixture into the bowl with the whole-wheat flour mixture, and stir until smooth.

Begin to stir in the all-purpose flour, ½ cup at a time, until you can no longer stir the mixture with a spoon. Turn out the dough onto a clean, floured work surface and knead the dough for 5 minutes. Add more all-purpose flour as you knead to prevent the dough from sticking. When you have finished kneading, the dough should be soft, smooth, and will spring back when poked with a finger; you may not need to use all of the flour.

Place the kneaded dough back in the mixing bowl, cover it loosely with plastic, and allow it to rise for 1 hour, or until doubled in volume.

Punch down the dough, turn it out onto a clean, floured work surface, and divide it into 12 pieces. Shape each piece of dough into a small ball and place them on a large baking sheet covered with parchment paper. Allow the rolls to rise for 1 hour more, or until doubled in volume.

While the rolls are rising, preheat the oven to 375°F.

Bake for about 30 minutes, or until golden brown on top.

BUDGET BYTE Once these rolls are completely cool, transfer them to a gallon-size freezer bag. The rolls can be kept frozen for up to 3 months and can be warmed quickly in the microwave or thawed at room temperature.

Chef's Tip: For a glossy, golden-brown roll, lightly whisk an egg white and brush it onto the surface of the rolls before baking.

Naan

$

*Makes
9 pieces*

This recipe has gone viral since I first posted it on the website three years ago, and not without good reason. These light and fluffy flatbreads are perfect for sopping up stews and gravies, stuffing full of seasoned meat or vegetables, or even using as the base for mini pizzas. They have a uniquely tender texture and an amazing sourdough-esque flavor. I have yet to meet anyone who hasn't gobbled up the whole batch within days—but if you can't, they also freeze well.

INGREDIENTS

2 teaspoons active dry or instant yeast

1 teaspoon sugar

½ cup warm water

3 cups all-purpose flour

½ teaspoon salt

2 tablespoons vegetable oil

⅓ cup plain yogurt

1 large egg

INSTRUCTIONS

In a small bowl, combine the yeast, sugar, and warm water. Stir until the yeast has dissolved and let stand for 5 minutes, or until the yeast becomes thick and frothy on top.

In a large bowl, stir together 1 cup of the flour and the salt until well combined.

Once the yeast is frothy, whisk in the oil, yogurt, and egg. Pour the yeast mixture into the bowl with the flour and salt and stir until smooth.

Add more flour, ½ cup at a time, until you can no longer stir the mixture with a spoon. Turn out the dough onto a clean, floured work surface. Knead the dough for 3 minutes, adding more flour as you knead to prevent the dough from sticking. When you have finished kneading it, the dough should be soft, smooth, and no longer sticky; you may not need to use all of the flour.

Return the dough to the mixing bowl, cover it loosely with plastic, and let it rise for 1 hour, or until doubled in volume.

Punch down the dough and divide it into 9 equal pieces. Shape each piece of dough into a ball.

Heat a heavy-bottomed skillet over medium heat. Press a ball of dough down into a flattened disc and then use a rolling pin to roll it out into a circle 6 inches in diameter. Repeat with the remaining dough balls. Dust each dough disc lightly with flour to keep it from sticking to the hot skillet.

Add 1 dough disc at a time to the skillet and cook for 1 to 2 minutes, or until golden brown on the bottom. Use tongs to flip the disc and cook until golden brown on the opposite side, 1 to 2 minutes more. Bubbles should form in the dough as it cooks. If not, raise the heat under the skillet slightly.

Repeat with the remaining dough discs. Pile the cooked naan on a clean plate as they come off the skillet and cover them with a clean, dry towel to keep them warm.

 BUDGET BYTE To store this bread, allow it to fully cool to room temperature, place it in a zip-top bag, and keep it refrigerated for up to 1 week or frozen for up to 3 months.

 Chef's Tip: For a more decadent naan, try oiling the skillet instead of dusting the raw dough with flour. This will produce a texture more reminiscent of fry bread. Once cooked, the naan can also be brushed with butter or ghee.

Italian Breadsticks

Makes 24

Say good-bye to bland, rock-hard breadsticks that cut open the roof of your mouth. These herb-infused breadsticks are chewy on the inside and perfectly crisp on the outside. Their long, thin shape makes them fun to eat and perfect for dipping into any sauce. Get the kids involved with this one, because these breadsticks are super fun to make!

INGREDIENTS

½ cup warm water

1 teaspoon active dry or instant yeast

1½ cups all-purpose flour

½ teaspoon salt

½ tablespoon Italian seasoning blend

1 tablespoon sugar

1 tablespoon olive oil

¼ cup yellow cornmeal

INSTRUCTIONS

In a small bowl, combine the warm water and yeast. Stir to dissolve the yeast and let stand for 5 minutes, or until the yeast becomes thick and frothy on top.

In a large bowl, combine ½ cup of the flour, the salt, and Italian seasoning blend and stir until evenly combined.

Stir the sugar and olive oil into the yeast mixture. Pour the yeast mixture into the bowl with the flour and salt. Stir until smooth.

Add more flour, ½ cup at a time, until you can no longer stir the mixture with a spoon. Turn out the dough onto a floured surface and knead for about 3 minutes, adding more flour as necessary to keep the dough from sticking. Place the kneaded dough back in the mixing bowl, cover it loosely with plastic wrap, and let it rise for 1 hour, or until doubled in volume.

Punch down the dough, turn it out onto a clean, floured work surface, and shape it into a 4-by-12-inch rectangle. Using a pizza cutter or dough scraper, cut the dough into 24 strips, about 4 inches long and ½ inch wide. Sprinkle a little of the cornmeal on the work surface, roll each strip of dough in the cornmeal, and then stretch it into a 12-inch-long rope.

Line a baking sheet with parchment paper. Place the dough strips on the parchment paper and let rise for 30 minutes.

While the dough is rising, preheat the oven to 400°F.

Bake the breadsticks for 15 to 18 minutes, or until golden brown in color. Serve warm or let cool to room temperature.

Four

DRESSINGS, DIPS & SAUCES

Dressing, dips, and sauces are where a meal comes to life. They convert boring pasta, meat, and vegetables into something unique and flavorful. If you have an arsenal of dressings, dips, and sauces under your belt, you can always whip up something special. And because homemade dressings and sauces don't contain fillers or flavorless bulking agents that dilute their taste, you'll find yourself needing to use far less on your food.

Basic Hummus *62*

Quick Salsa *64*

Best Bean Dip *66*

The "Real Deal" Chip Dip *68*

Balsamic Tomato Bruschetta *69*

Creamy Cilantro-Lime
Dressing *71*

Lighter Ranch Dressing *72*

Creamy Balsamic Dressing *73*

Sesame-Ginger Dressing *74*

Easy Meat Sauce *76*

Red Enchilada Sauce *77*

Basic Hummus

*Makes
2¹/₂ cups*

I can't fully express my love for hummus. It runs deep, very deep. Hummus is creamy, garlicky, bright, and lemony perfection. You can use it as a dip for pita bread, crackers, or vegetables, but it can also be used as a spread on sandwiches, wraps, or even pizza. Once you realize how effortless it is to make, you'll never buy one of those expensive tubs from the grocery store again.

INGREDIENTS

1 (15-ounce) can chickpeas,
    drained and rinsed

2 tablespoons olive oil

¼ cup lemon juice

¼ cup tahini (sesame seed paste;
    see Chef's Tip, at right)

1 clove garlic

½ teaspoon salt

⅛ teaspoon ground cumin

INSTRUCTIONS

In the bowl of a food processor or in a blender, combine the chickpeas, olive oil, lemon juice, tahini, garlic, salt, and cumin and process or blend until smooth. Add ¼ to ½ cup of water to help smooth out the mixture and to obtain your desired consistency. If you are using a blender, you'll likely need a little more water than if you are using a food processor.

Variations

- **Jalapeño-Cilantro Hummus**—Remove the seeds from a jalapeño and add it to the hummus along with a handful of fresh cilantro. Process until smooth.
- **Roasted Red Pepper Hummus**—Add 1 whole roasted red pepper (from a jar) to the hummus. Process until smooth.

- **Green Onion & Parsley Hummus**—Add 3 trimmed green onions and a handful of fresh parsley leaves to the hummus. Process until smooth.

 Chef's Tip: Tahini, a paste made from pureed sesame seeds, is the key to making an authentic-tasting hummus. In grocery stores, tahini is usually sold in the international foods section, near other Mediterranean ingredients like kalamata olives, artichoke hearts, and roasted red peppers, although it can sometimes be found near the peanut butter.

Quick Salsa $

Makes 3 cups

I'm a total salsa fiend, and when I want it I've *got* to have it, so having a good homemade salsa recipe is an absolute must. This is my favorite recipe, which is a cross between a cooked salsa and a fresh salsa. Canned tomatoes give the salsa a deeper, richer flavor, and fresh red onion, garlic, cilantro, and jalapeño add a bright kick. When I have this salsa in my refrigerator, I find any excuse I can to add it to my meal. Eggs, chicken, rice—they're all better with a spoonful of salsa on top! If you want an extra-spicy salsa, leave in some of the jalapeño seeds.

INGREDIENTS

1 clove garlic

1 small red onion, quartered

1 medium jalapeño, stemmed and seeded

1 (28-ounce) can whole or diced tomatoes

½ bunch fresh cilantro, leaves only, plus more as needed

1 teaspoon salt, plus more as needed

½ tablespoon sugar

2 tablespoons olive oil

Juice of 1 medium lime, plus more as needed

INSTRUCTIONS

In the bowl of a food processor, combine the garlic, onion, and jalapeño. Pulse the mixture until the ingredients are finely chopped.

Add the canned tomatoes and their juices, the cilantro, salt, sugar, olive oil, and lime juice and pulse the mixture until it reaches the desired consistency (longer for a smooth salsa, or less for a chunkier salsa). Taste and add additional salt, cilantro, or lime juice until the flavor is to your liking.

Chef's Tip: For an extra-chunky salsa, or if you don't have a food processor, simply chop the ingredients by hand and stir them together.

Best Bean Dip

"Bean dip? Really?"

Yeah, I know. Bean dip is so boring, right? I thought so, too, until I realized that I was reaching into my fridge to eat this three times a day and dipping *anything* I could into it (seriously, though, popcorn is great for dipping when you don't have any chips or pita around). Granted, I *love* refried beans, but when they're jazzed up like this, they're a whole new beast. Eat this dip as a light meal with some whole-grain pita, serve it at a party with chips, or use it as a filling for quick-and-simple bean burritos.

INGREDIENTS

1 tablespoon olive oil

1 medium jalapeño, stemmed and seeded

2 cloves garlic, minced

1 (31-ounce) can refried beans

1 (14.5-ounce) can diced tomatoes with chiles (see Chef's Tip, below)

1 teaspoon ground cumin

½ teaspoon chili powder

INSTRUCTIONS

In a large skillet, heat the olive oil over medium heat. Add the jalapeño and garlic and sauté for 2 to 3 minutes, or until softened. Add the refried beans, tomatoes with their juices, cumin, and chili powder and stir until combined. Continue to cook until heated through, 5 to 7 minutes, then serve.

 Chef's Tip: If you can't find canned tomatoes with chiles, you can purchase the two ingredients separately; use 1 (15-ounce) can diced tomatoes and 1 (4-ounce) can mild green chiles.

Chef's Tip: For an extra-rich bean dip, add ½ to 1 cup shredded Monterey Jack or cheddar to the bean-tomato mixture in the skillet and stir until melted.

The "Real Deal" Chip Dip $

Makes
1 cup

Your chips deserve better than white, gloppy modified cornstarch and artificial flavorings. Show them you love them by whipping up a batch of this homemade chip dip. It takes just a few short minutes to have fresh, zesty dip that is perfect for chips, vegetables, and crackers alike. The best part? You control the salt, you control the flavor, and you know every single ingredient that goes into it. Oh, not to mention it's *also* less expensive than store-bought dips and packet mixes.

INGREDIENTS

1 cup light or regular sour cream

2 tablespoons mayonnaise

1 teaspoon lemon juice

⅛ teaspoon garlic powder

¾ teaspoon salt

Freshly cracked black pepper

⅛ teaspoon dried dill (optional)

2 green onions, thinly sliced

INSTRUCTIONS

In a small bowl, combine the sour cream, mayonnaise, lemon juice, garlic powder, salt, cracked pepper to taste, and dill, if using, and stir until well combined.

Stir the sliced green onions into the dip. Serve immediately or refrigerate for 30 minutes to allow the flavors to blend.

 BUDGET BYTE Mayonnaise adds extra richness and a creamy flavor, but if you don't have it on hand, the dip will still be fantastic without.

 Chef's Tip: If you're watching your fat or calorie intake, try substituting high-quality nonfat Greek yogurt for the sour cream.

Balsamic Tomato Bruschetta $$

Although bruschetta is usually thought of as an appetizer, I could make a meal out of it. Give me a good loaf of French bread and a bowl of bruschetta topping and that's all I need in the world. Traditionally, bruschetta is toasted slices of bread with various toppings, but this tomato topping can also be used on chicken, fish, or even eggs. It's so good you may even want to just eat it with a spoon! I cut costs on this bruschetta by using dried basil instead of fresh, but brighten it up with fresh parsley, which is much less expensive than basil.

Makes 2 cups

INGREDIENTS

¼ cup olive oil

4 cloves garlic, minced

4 medium Roma tomatoes, diced

½ tablespoon dried basil

Freshly cracked black pepper

1 tablespoon balsamic vinegar

¼ teaspoon salt

Handful of fresh parsley

1 French baguette, sliced crosswise into ½-inch pieces

INSTRUCTIONS

In a medium skillet, heat the olive oil over medium-low heat. Add the garlic and cook, stirring, for 5 minutes, or until the garlic has softened but not browned. Remove the pan from the heat and let the garlic cool slightly.

In a bowl, combine the tomatoes, basil, a generous dose of cracked pepper, the balsamic vinegar, and the salt. Pull the parsley leaves from the stems and give them a rough chop. Add the parsley and stir to combine.

Using a spoon, transfer the garlic and about half of the olive oil from the skillet to the bowl with the tomatoes. Stir everything together.

Return the skillet to the stovetop over medium heat. Toast the baguette slices in the skillet with the remaining garlic-infused oil. Serve the toasted baguette slices topped with spoonfuls of the tomato topping.

Chef's Tip: The juices that collect in the bottom of the bowl of bruschetta topping are also wonderful for soaking up with fresh bread. I like to leave some of the baguette slices untoasted, as it soaks up the liquid more readily.

Creamy Cilantro-Lime Dressing $$

Oh, how I love this dressing! Super tangy, a little creamy, and absolutely bursting with freshness. It whips up in just a few minutes and can be used for much more than just salads. I love dipping my Beef & Bean Taquitos (page 150) and Cumin-Lime Sweet Potato Sticks (page 198) into it, but it would also go great poured over a grilled skirt steak or even my Cumin, Lime & Chickpea Salad (page 85).

*Makes
³/₄ cup*

INGREDIENTS

1 clove garlic, minced

2 tablespoons fresh lime juice (from
    ½ medium lime)

¼ cup olive oil

¼ cup sour cream

½ teaspoon salt

½ tablespoon honey

¼ bunch fresh cilantro, leaves only

INSTRUCTIONS

In a blender, combine the garlic, lime juice, olive oil, sour cream, salt, and honey. Blend until smooth.

Add the cilantro and blend briefly or until the leaves are in small pieces and the mixture is light green in color. The dressing will keep in an airtight container in the refrigerator for up to 1 week.

 Chef's Tip: To get the most juice from your lime, roll it on the counter while applying pressure before cutting it open. Twist a spoon into the flesh to extract as much juice as possible.

Lighter Ranch Dressing $$

Makes 1¹/₂ cups

Once you realize how quick and easy it is to make your own ranch dressing, you'll probably never buy it again. This version has such an amazingly light, fresh, and tangy flavor, yet has a much lower fat content than traditional ranch dressings. Ranch dressing is becoming a universal condiment, and it's easy to see why. Not only is it great for salads, but it also works as a spread on sandwiches and wraps, or as a dip for vegetables (fresh *or* roasted), like my Firecracker Cauliflower (page 207).

INGREDIENTS

½ cup low-fat buttermilk

¾ cup low-fat plain yogurt

¼ cup mayonnaise

½ tablespoon lemon juice

½ teaspoon salt, plus more as needed

½ teaspoon garlic powder

Freshly cracked black pepper

1 green onion, thinly sliced

Handful of fresh parsley, leaves only, chopped

INSTRUCTIONS

In a bowl, whisk together the buttermilk, yogurt, mayonnaise, lemon juice, salt, garlic powder, and pepper to taste.

Stir the green onion and parsley into the dressing. Cover and refrigerate the mixture for at least 30 minutes to allow the flavors to blend. Taste and adjust the salt, if desired, before serving.

Chef's Tip: While I do like to cut some fat, I advise against cutting it all out. Fat plays an important role in creating texture and balancing the dressing's flavor. Real buttermilk is key to getting that authentic ranch flavor, so don't be tempted to use shortcuts, like adding lemon juice or vinegar to milk.

Creamy Balsamic Dressing $$

A simple vinaigrette is probably one of the easiest things you'll ever make—just throw all of the ingredients in a blender and press go. Making this luscious, creamy vinaigrette is just as simple and tastes so good that you'll be tempted to drink it with a spoon. Forget the store-bought vinaigrette because this one only takes five minutes to make and has such big flavor that you'll only need to use a splash. Now you can have fresh, gourmet dressing at every meal.

*Makes
1 cup*

INGREDIENTS

1 clove garlic, minced

¼ cup olive oil

¼ cup mayonnaise

¼ cup plain yogurt

¼ cup balsamic vinegar

1 tablespoon Dijon mustard

1 teaspoon sugar

½ teaspoon salt, plus more as needed

½ teaspoon dried oregano

INSTRUCTIONS

In a blender, combine the garlic, olive oil, mayonnaise, yogurt, vinegar, mustard, sugar, salt, and oregano and blend until smooth. Taste the dressing and adjust the salt as needed. Store the dressing in an airtight container in the refrigerator for up to 1 week.

 Chef's Tip: While this dressing will work with reduced-fat mayonnaise and low-fat yogurt, I wouldn't suggest using fat-free versions. The fat is needed not only to balance the flavors but also to achieve the correct consistency.

Sesame-Ginger Dressing $$

Makes
1¼ cups

You know those gourmet salad dressings they sell refrigerated in the produce section at the grocery store? The kind that try to justify their hefty price tag with exotic-sounding ingredients like toasted sesame oil and ginger? Well, once I discovered that I could make the same thing at home in about sixty seconds and for pennies on the dollar, my world changed. I went from looking longingly at those grocery store dressings to throwing a smug side-eye, as if to say, "I'm onto you."

This dressing is sweet, creamy, and rich, with a little sassy bite. I love it over salads, but it also goes great with fresh vegetables like cucumber or carrots, or even cold soba noodles.

INGREDIENTS

2 cloves garlic, roughly chopped

½ cup vegetable oil

¼ cup rice vinegar

2 tablespoons soy sauce

3 tablespoons honey

1 tablespoon tahini (sesame seed paste)

½ teaspoon toasted sesame oil

4-inch piece fresh ginger, peeled

INSTRUCTIONS

In a blender, combine the garlic, vegetable oil, vinegar, soy sauce, honey, tahini, and sesame oil.

Using a small-holed cheese grater or a Microplane, grate the ginger straight into the blender so that none of its juices are lost.

Blend the dressing until smooth. Serve immediately or refrigerate in an airtight container for up to 1 week.

BUDGET BYTE Fresh ginger can be found in the produce department. You don't need to buy the whole root. Simply break off the amount that you need, just as you might divide a bunch of bananas when you only want a few.

 BUDGET BYTE Rice vinegar, tahini, and toasted sesame oil may seem like foreign ingredients, but all three are staples in Asian cooking and can be found in most major grocery stores today.

Easy Meat Sauce

$$

Makes
4 cups

This is my go-to quick red sauce. The Italian sausage has so many herbs and spices built right in that you barely need to add anything else to make a super-flavorful sauce. In less than thirty minutes you'll have a thick, rich sauce that you could probably pass off as a secret family recipe. For an extra-meaty sauce, use a full pound of sausage. Otherwise, just use a half pound, as I have here, and freeze the rest for use in another recipe.

INGREDIENTS

1 tablespoon olive oil

1 small yellow onion, diced

2 cloves garlic, minced

½ pound Italian sausage (hot or mild)

1 (28-ounce) can crushed tomatoes

1 (6-ounce) can tomato paste

½ teaspoon dried basil

½ teaspoon dried oregano

1 tablespoon sugar

½ teaspoon salt

INSTRUCTIONS

In a large saucepan, heat the oil over medium heat. Add the onion and garlic and cook until the onions are tender and translucent, 3 to 5 minutes.

If your Italian sausage is in a casing, squeeze it out of the casing. Discard the casing and add the sausage to the pan. Continue to cook until the sausage is thoroughly browned, breaking it up with the side of a wooden spoon as it cooks.

Add the crushed tomatoes and stir to loosen any browned bits on the bottom of the pot. Add the tomato paste, basil, oregano, sugar, and salt and stir until combined. Continue to cook until heated through. Taste the sauce and adjust the seasoning, if desired. Serve hot over your favorite pasta, or let cool and store in an airtight container in the refrigerator for 5 to 7 days.

Red Enchilada Sauce

I used to think that making enchilada sauce would require special dried peppers, hours at the stove, and living in Central America for at least six months (you know, so you could claim authenticity). I mean, why else were they charging over two dollars for a little can of this stuff? Imagine my surprise when I finally tried to make it at home and found that not only was my result ten times more flavorful than the canned version, but it took less than ten minutes to make, and used only pantry staples. It changed my life. Now I use this sauce to drench enchiladas and burritos, as well as to spice up rice and pasta dishes, like my Loaded Enchilada Pasta (page 104). So go ahead and kick the can (of enchilada sauce).

INGREDIENTS

2 tablespoons vegetable oil

2 tablespoons all-purpose flour

2 tablespoons chili powder

¼ cup tomato paste

½ teaspoon ground cumin

½ teaspoon garlic powder

¼ teaspoon cayenne pepper

½ teaspoon salt, plus more as needed

INSTRUCTIONS

Add the vegetable oil, flour, and chili powder to a medium saucepan and place the pan over medium heat. Whisk the ingredients together. Cook until the mixture begins to bubble, then continue to cook and whisk for 1 minute more.

Add the tomato paste, cumin, garlic powder, cayenne pepper, and 2 cups of water and whisk until smooth. Allow the mixture to come to a simmer, at which point it will thicken slightly. Whisk in the salt; taste the sauce and add more salt, if desired. Remove the pan from the heat, and serve.

 Chef's Tip: For extra flavor, replace the water with chicken broth. Because most store-bought broths are heavily salted, adjust the salt added in the last step as necessary.

Five

SALADS

Salads are all about creating a mélange of flavors, textures, and colors. The more variety and contrast, the more fun they are to eat. They're a great way to incorporate vegetables and nutrients into your diet and can serve double duty as either a side dish or a light meal.

Unfortunately, salads can easily gobble up your budget when you get carried away with fancy or extravagant toppings or let uneaten vegetables go limp. For healthy and affordable salads, keep it simple. Choose vegetables that are in season, and use a light hand with nuts, dried fruit, and cheese.

Super-Crunch Salad   *80*

Summer Melon Salad   *82*

Lentil & Feta Salad   *83*

Cumin, Lime & Chickpea Salad   *85*

Vinaigrette Slaw with Feta   *86*

Apple Dijon Kale Salad   *87*

Tomato & White Bean Salad   *89*

Easy Asian Slaw   *90*

Mango, Jalapeño & Quinoa Salad   *91*

Greek Chopped Salad   *93*

Dijon Potato & Green Bean Salad   *94*

Southwest Chicken Salad   *96*

Super-Crunch Salad $$

*Serves
6 to 8*

This is my superhero green salad. Unlike most green salads, it stays fresh and crunchy for almost a week. If that's not a superpower, then I don't know what is! The rainbow of colors and super-crunchy texture make this salad a little less boring than your average side salad. You can prepare all the ingredients ahead of time and then quickly assemble the salad just before each meal. While this salad pairs well with a variety of different dressing types, I love it with my Creamy Balsamic Dressing (page 73) the best.

INGREDIENTS

1 small head red cabbage, quartered
   and cored

3 medium carrots

1 (16-ounce) container baby spinach

1 cup sliced almonds

1 cup dried cranberries

Dressing of your choice

INSTRUCTIONS

Slice the cabbage thinly. Store the thinly sliced cabbage in a large resealable food container or zip-top bag.

Use a vegetable peeler to shave the carrots into thin, crunchy strips. Store the carrot strips in a large resealable food container or zip-top bag.

To prepare each salad serving, create a bed of baby spinach and top it with a handful of sliced cabbage, carrots strips, and about 2 tablespoons each of sliced almonds and dried cranberries. Top the salad with your favorite dressing. To keep the ingredients fresh and crunchy, wait until just before serving to add the dressing.

BUDGET BYTE Baby spinach packaged in large, resealable plastic tubs lasts twice as long as spinach packaged in nonresealable bags. If it looks like you won't be able to eat all of it before it goes bad, spinach can be frozen and added to smoothies for a hidden nutritional punch.

BUDGET BYTE Find the smallest head of cabbage possible because once it is sliced, the volume of cabbage is always much more than anticipated.

Summer Melon Salad $

Serves 6

In midsummer, when melons are at their peak, their flavor (and price) can't be beat. This simple salad allows the melon's natural flavor to shine through, while mint and lime add a hint of unique flavor. It's a wonderful treat for breakfast, a light side for lunch, or even a healthy dessert after dinner.

Mint is not only one of the least expensive herbs to buy, but it also grows like wildfire. Ask around to see if anyone you know grows it, or try planting some yourself! It requires almost no maintenance and will provide you with more mint than your mojito habit can handle!

INGREDIENTS

1 large cantaloupe or honeydew melon, halved and seeded

Juice of 1 medium lime

1 tablespoon honey

2 to 3 sprigs fresh mint

Salt (optional)

INSTRUCTIONS

Cut the melon into wedges. Using a small knife, remove the rind and cut the flesh into small cubes. Place the cubed melon in a large bowl.

In a small bowl, stir together the lime juice and honey. Pour the honey-lime mixture over the melon.

Pull the mint leaves from their stems and roughly chop them. Add the mint to the melon and toss to combine and coat in the honey-lime mixture.

Serve the salad with a pinch of salt over each bowl, if desired.

 BUDGET BYTE Save this recipe for when melons are at their peak. The rest of the year, melons tend to be overpriced and have lackluster flavor.

Lentil & Feta Salad

Serves 4

I love lentils because they have all the healthy goodness of beans without the hassle of presoaking or hours of boiling. This easy Mediterranean salad packs a *huge* flavor punch and can be eaten either as a side dish or stuffed into a pita with fresh tomatoes for a quick vegetarian lunch. I love having hearty salads like this in my fridge to eat all week long.

INGREDIENTS

1 cup brown lentils

¼ bunch fresh flat-leaf parsley, leaves only, roughly chopped

1 clove garlic, minced

2 tablespoons olive oil

1 tablespoon lemon juice

½ teaspoon salt

2 ounces feta cheese, crumbled

INSTRUCTIONS

Sift through the lentils and remove any stones or other debris. Fill a medium saucepan with water, cover, and bring to a boil over high heat. Add the lentils and return the water to a boil. Reduce the heat to medium-low and simmer, uncovered, for about 15 minutes, or until the lentils are tender but not mushy.

Drain the lentils in a colander and place them in the refrigerator to cool while you prepare the rest of the salad.

In a medium bowl, combine the parsley, garlic, olive oil, lemon juice, salt, and feta. Add the cooled cooked lentils and stir to combine. Serve immediately or refrigerate until ready to eat.

Chef's Tip: All lentils are not created equal. Brown lentils cook quickly, while green or French lentils take up to 45 minutes to cook. If you're unsure of whether you have brown or green lentils, check the cooking time on the back of the package. Look for lentils that suggest a 15- to 20-minute cooking time. Red, orange, and yellow lentils lose their shape and become mushy when cooked, making them not well suited for this salad.

Cumin, Lime & Chickpea Salad $

This salad is great whenever your meal needs a jolt of flavor and freshness. Lime and cilantro taste like sunshine in your mouth while small bits of red onion and garlic give each bite a major zing. Buttery chickpeas and earthy cumin help ground the flavor, making for a well-rounded and super-hearty salad. Want to try a creamy version? Substitute my Creamy Cilantro-Lime Dressing (page 71) for the simple lime and cumin dressing below.

Serves 6

INGREDIENTS

2 (15-ounce) cans chickpeas, drained and rinsed

½ medium red onion, finely diced

½ bunch fresh cilantro, leaves only, roughly chopped

2 cloves garlic, minced

Juice of 1 medium lime

2 tablespoons olive oil

1 teaspoon ground cumin

⅛ teaspoon cayenne pepper

¼ teaspoon salt

INSTRUCTIONS

In a large bowl, combine the chickpeas, onion, cilantro, and garlic and stir to combine.

In a small bowl, combine the lime juice, olive oil, cumin, cayenne pepper, and salt, and stir briefly to combine. Pour the dressing over the salad and toss until everything is well mixed and coated in the dressing.

 BUDGET BYTE To get the most juice from your lime, roll it on the counter while applying pressure before cutting it open. Twist a spoon into the flesh to extract as much juice as possible.

Vinaigrette Slaw with Feta $$

Serves 8

My friend Jenni told me about this insanely simple yet super-flavorful salad, and I've been addicted ever since. With just a few ingredients, this salad is a cinch to prepare and has a bold flavor that pairs well with almost any type of cuisine. I love the way the dressing soaks into the cabbage, making the salad more flavorful as the days go by.

INGREDIENTS

½ small head green cabbage, cored

½ small head red cabbage, cored

4 ounces feta cheese, crumbled

1 cup Caesar dressing

INSTRUCTIONS

Thinly slice the green and red cabbages. Place the sliced cabbage in a large bowl and toss to combine.

Sprinkle the feta cheese over the cabbage and drizzle with Caesar dressing. Stir to coat the cabbage in the dressing and cheese. Serve immediately or refrigerate and allow the cabbage to marinate in the dressing. It will keep for up to 5 days.

BUDGET BYTE Shred the unused halves of the cabbages and freeze the shredded cabbage for later use in soup, stir-fry, or egg rolls. Frozen cabbage will soften slightly, so it's best to use it in cooked dishes rather than fresh salads.

Chef's Tip: If you want faster prep and no leftovers, use preshredded cabbage (or coleslaw mix) or just one head of red cabbage rather than half of each color.

Apple Dijon Kale Salad $

Kale is my favorite salad green because it's *so* hearty and filling that you're never left hungry afterward. It's like a meal in and of itself. Granny Smith apples add a crisp crunch and sweet-tart flavor that is echoed in the tart apple cider vinaigrette and sweet raisins. A few walnuts add even more crunch and a mild creaminess that helps ground the bright flavors and fill your belly. Every bite has flavor and texture to be discovered, so you'll never get bored. Want something even more extravagant? Try crumbling some creamy goat cheese on top.

Serves 4

INGREDIENTS

1 clove garlic, minced

⅓ cup olive oil

¼ cup apple cider vinegar

1½ tablespoons Dijon mustard

¼ teaspoon salt, plus more as needed

Freshly cracked black pepper

1 bunch kale, stemmed

1 medium Granny Smith apple,
    cored and chopped

½ cup chopped walnuts

¼ cup raisins

INSTRUCTIONS

In a blender, combine the garlic, olive oil, vinegar, mustard, salt, and 10 to 15 grinds of a pepper mill. Blend the ingredients until smooth. Taste and adjust the salt and pepper, if desired.

Tear the kale leaves into small, bite-size pieces. Place the torn leaves in a colander and rinse well with cool water. Allow as much excess water to drain away as possible.

Place the kale leaves in a large bowl and top with the apple, walnuts, and raisins. Pour the apple cider vinaigrette over the top and toss to coat.

BUDGET BYTE The ingredients for this salad are very hearty and stand up to refrigeration well. The acid in the apple cider vinegar will help prevent the apples from browning and will slowly soften the kale leaves, making them even more delicious as the days go on. Unlike most green salads, this salad will keep, pre-dressed, for 3 to 4 days in the refrigerator.

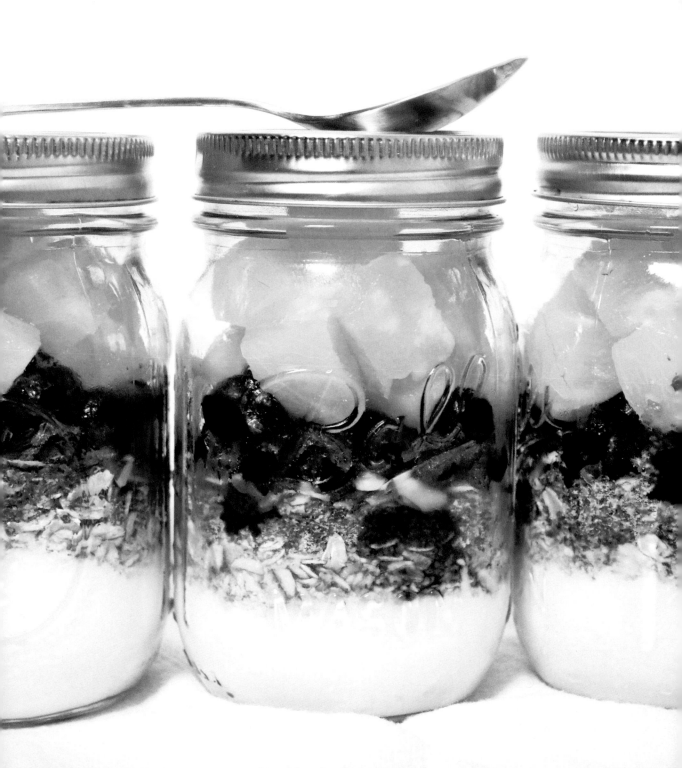

Breakfast Parfaits, page 22

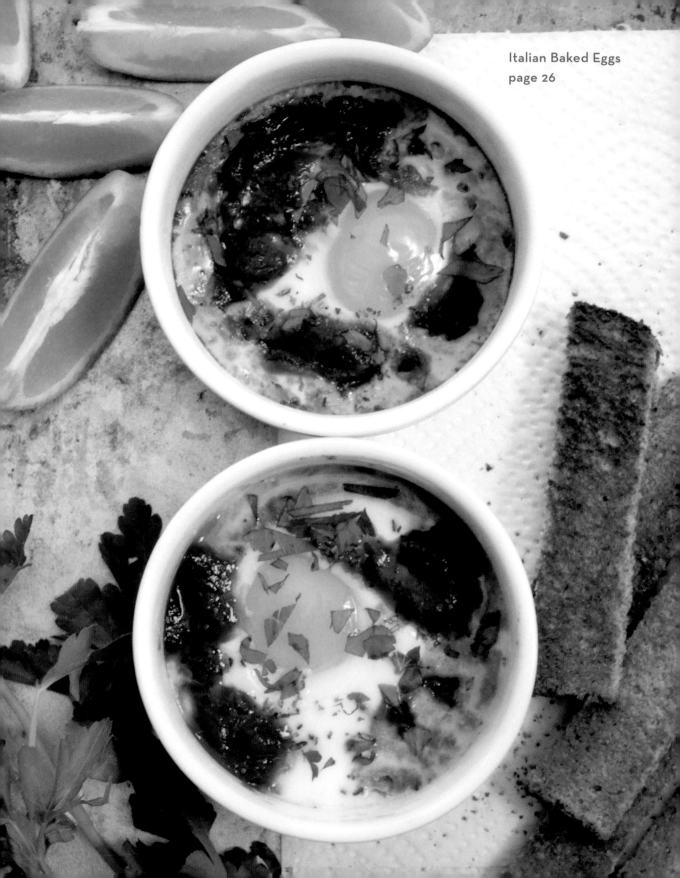

Italian Baked Eggs
page 26

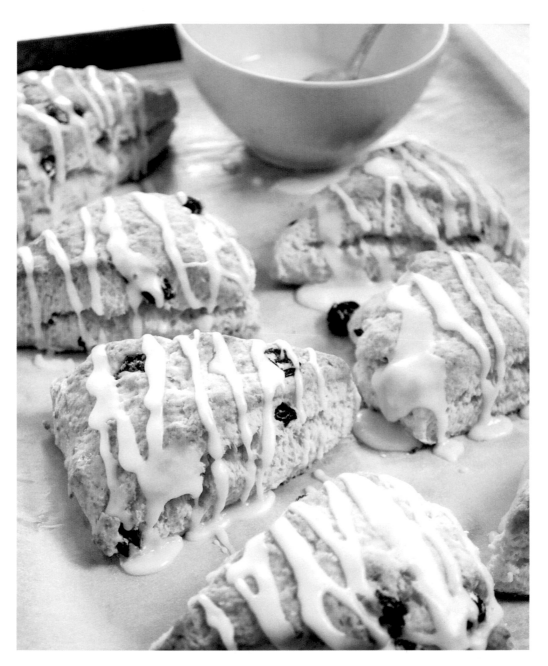

Iced Orange-Cranberry Scones

page 33

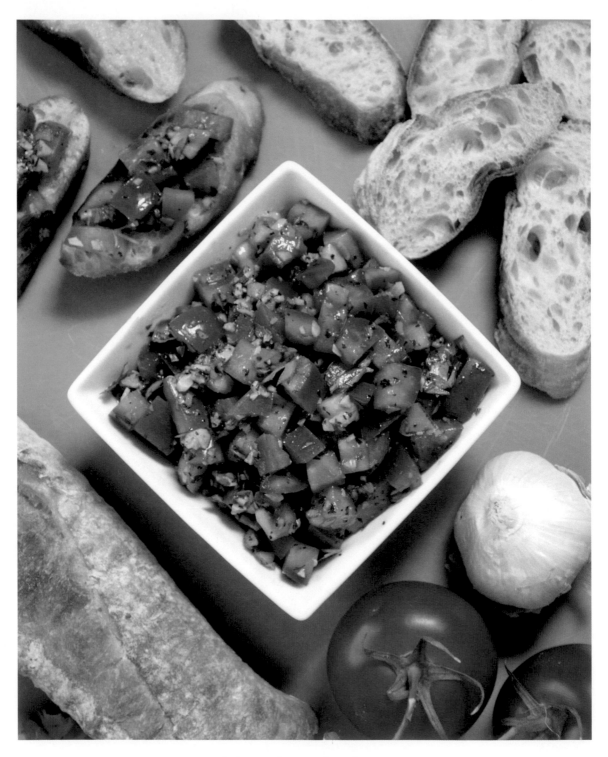

Balsamic Tomato Bruschetta

page 69

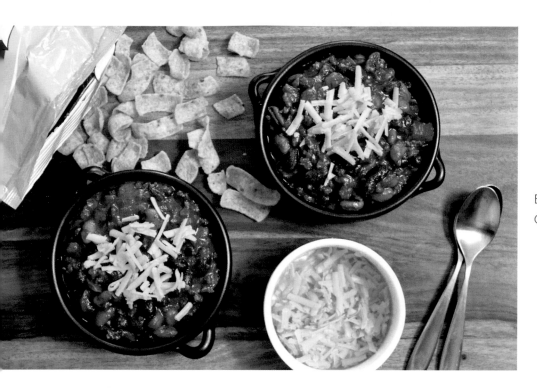

Better-Than-Mom's
Chili, page 134

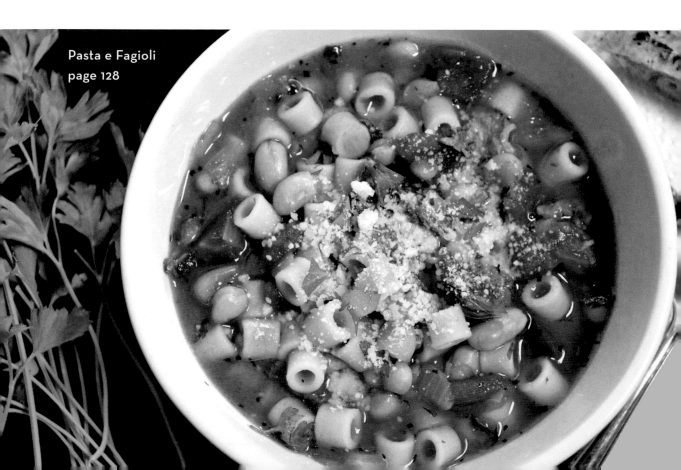

Pasta e Fagioli
page 128

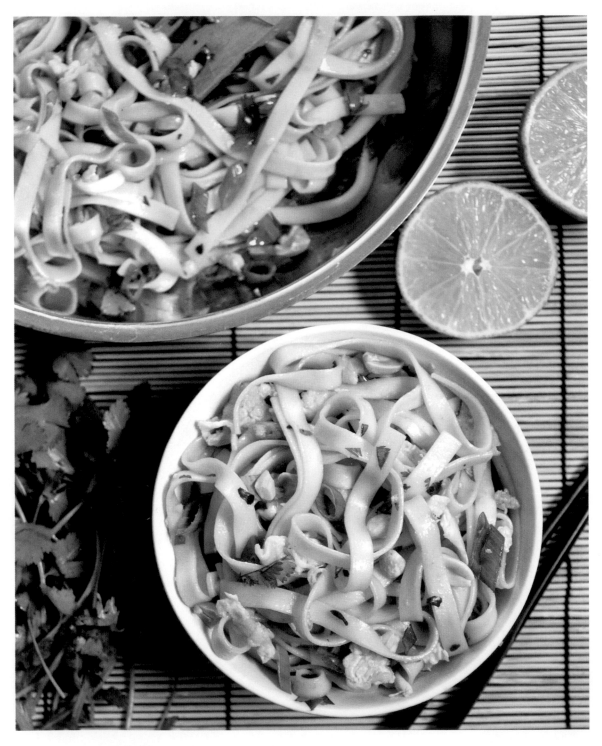

Easy Pad Thai

page 112

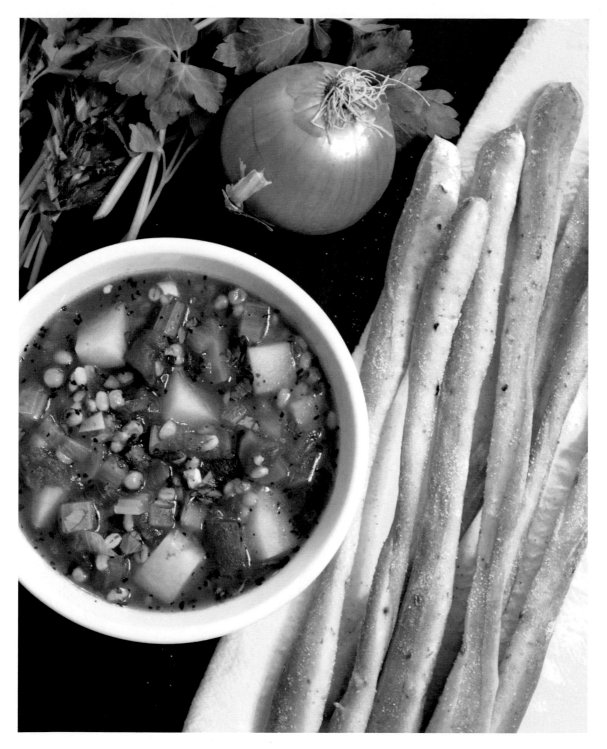

Hearty Vegetable & Barley Soup, page 136
with Italian Breadsticks, page 58

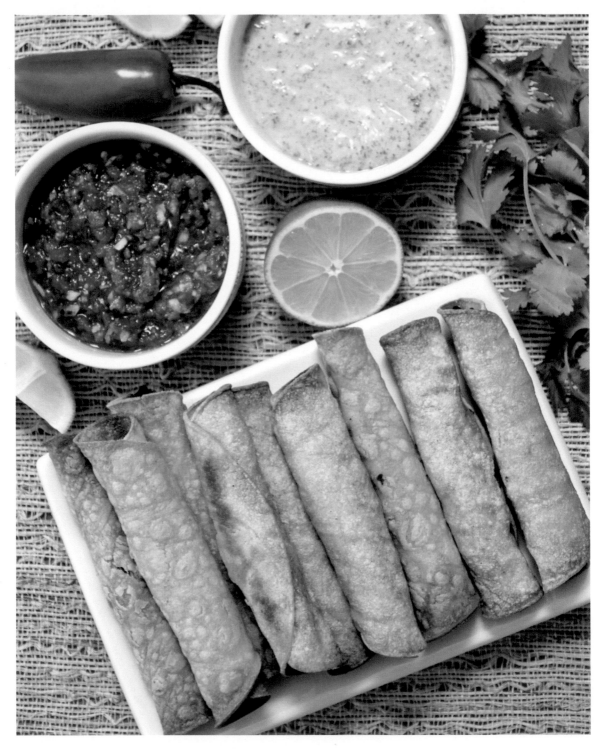

Beef & Bean Taquitos, page 150
with Creamy Cilantro-Lime Dressing, page 71

Tomato & White Bean Salad $

This quick salad reminds me of a classic tomato sandwich. Tangy, fresh tomatoes are perfectly balanced with creamy white beans, and a few green onions provide a fresh kick. A simple dressing of olive oil, salt, and pepper really allows the flavor of the tomatoes to shine through. Serve this salad alongside sandwiches or grilled meats for a light summertime meal.

Serves 4

INGREDIENTS

1 (15-ounce) can Great Northern beans, drained and rinsed

1 large tomato, diced

2 green onions, thinly sliced

1 tablespoon olive oil

½ teaspoon salt, plus more as needed

Freshly cracked black pepper

INSTRUCTIONS

In a medium bowl, combine the beans, tomato, and green onions.

Drizzle the olive oil over the salad, sprinkle it with salt, and add some pepper. Stir to combine, taste, and adjust the salt and pepper to your liking.

BUDGET BYTE For the most flavor and best price, prepare this salad when tomatoes are at the height of their season!

Chef's Tip: If you prefer a more complex flavor, try stirring chopped fresh or dried basil into the finished salad.

Easy Asian Slaw $

Serves 4

Asian slaw is a light, tangy alternative to traditional mayo-heavy American slaws. Although slaw is usually eaten as a side dish, it can be used for so much more. Slaw makes a wonderfully crunchy topping to sandwiches, like my Teriyaki Chicken Sliders (page 162), or it can be stuffed into a wrap with grilled chicken, mandarin oranges, and sliced almonds. Use it as a bed for grilled shrimp or salmon, or stuff them all into a tortilla for an Asian-inspired taco.

INGREDIENTS

1 (10-ounce) bag shredded cabbage or coleslaw mix (about 4 cups)

2 green onions, sliced

1 medium carrot

1 tablespoon vegetable oil

1 tablespoon natural peanut butter

1½ tablespoons soy sauce

1 tablespoon rice vinegar

1 tablespoon brown sugar

1 tablespoon hot water

1 clove garlic

1-inch piece fresh ginger, peeled

INSTRUCTIONS

In a large bowl, combine the cabbage and the green onions. Using a large-holed cheese grater, shred the carrot into the bowl.

In a blender, combine the vegetable oil, peanut butter, soy sauce, vinegar, sugar, hot water, and garlic. Using a small-holed cheese grater or a Microplane, grate the ginger into the blender. Blend the dressing until smooth.

Pour the dressing over the vegetables in the bowl and stir to coat.

 Chef's Tip: To customize this salad, try adding other ingredients like edamame, dry ramen noodles, almonds, cilantro, or red bell peppers.

Mango, Jalapeño & Quinoa Salad $$

This light salad smells and tastes like a tropical breeze. It's slightly sweet, a little spicy, *Serves 4* and super fresh. But don't let the light flavor deceive you! Quinoa packs a real protein punch that will help keep you full for hours. It's the perfect light summer salad or side dish for fish or grilled chicken.

INGREDIENTS

1 cup quinoa

1½ cups chicken broth

¼ cup rice vinegar

1½ tablespoons sugar

½ teaspoon salt

⅛ teaspoon red pepper flakes

1 medium mango, peeled and cubed

½ bunch green onions, sliced

½ bunch cilantro, chopped

1 medium jalapeño, seeded and minced

INSTRUCTIONS

Rinse the quinoa well in a fine-mesh sieve. Alternatively, place the quinoa in a bowl of cool water, swish it around several times, and then carefully pour off as much water as possible. In a medium pot, combine the rinsed quinoa and chicken broth. Cover and bring to a boil over high heat. Reduce the heat to low and let simmer for 15 minutes. After 15 minutes, remove the pot from the heat and let it stand, covered and undisturbed, for 15 minutes more, then uncover and fluff the quinoa with a fork.

In a small bowl, combine the vinegar, sugar, salt, and red pepper flakes and stir until the sugar is mostly dissolved.

In a large bowl, combine the cooked quinoa, mango, green onions, cilantro, and jalapeño. Pour the vinegar dressing over the quinoa mixture and stir until well combined. Serve immediately or refrigerate until ready to eat.

BUDGET BYTE If mangoes are out of season or just not available at a reasonable price, try substituting fresh or canned pineapple.

 BUDGET BYTE Purchasing quinoa from bulk bins allows you to buy the exact amount that you need and often at a much lower price than prepackaged varieties.

Greek Chopped Salad $$

This is one of my favorite summertime salads because it takes advantage of all the summer vegetables when they are at their peak of freshness. Cucumber, tomato, green bell pepper, and onion make salads taste super fresh, while chickpeas give *oomph* and belly-filling power. A fresh, homemade vinaigrette tops it off along with a light sprinkle of feta cheese for a little salty contrast. Eat it as a side salad or stuff it into a pita for a light vegetarian lunch.

Serves 6

INGREDIENTS

1 medium cucumber, diced

1 medium tomato, diced

1 medium green bell pepper, diced

1 small red onion, diced

¼ bunch fresh flat-leaf parsley, leaves only, roughly chopped

1 (15-ounce) can chickpeas, drained and rinsed

2 ounces feta cheese, crumbled

1 (8-ounce) jar sliced banana peppers

¼ cup olive oil

2 tablespoons red wine vinegar

1 teaspoon dried oregano

¼ teaspoon salt

1 clove garlic

INSTRUCTIONS

In a large bowl, combine the cucumber, tomato, bell pepper, red onion, and parsley. Toss to combine. Add the chickpeas to the bowl, along with the feta and banana peppers.

In a blender, combine the olive oil, vinegar, oregano, salt, and garlic and blend until the garlic is minced and the dressing is evenly mixed.

Pour the dressing over the salad and toss to coat.

Dijon Potato & Green Bean Salad $

Potato salad is pure comfort. Starchy potatoes, creamy dressing, and just enough tang to keep you coming back for more . . . and more . . . and more. This version is a little bit lighter, with green beans added to balance out the starchy potatoes and a slightly lighter herbal Dijon dressing. It's comfort food with a *little* less guilt!

INGREDIENTS

2 pounds waxy potatoes, such as Yukon Gold, cut into 1-inch cubes

½ pound green beans

3 green onions

¼ cup mayonnaise

3 tablespoons Dijon mustard

½ teaspoon sugar

½ teaspoon dried thyme

¼ teaspoon salt

Freshly cracked black pepper

INSTRUCTIONS

Place the potatoes in a medium pot and add enough cold water to cover them by 1 inch. Cover the pot and bring the water to a boil over high heat.

Once the water reaches a boil, remove the lid and continue to boil for 5 to 7 minutes, or until the potatoes are very tender when pierced with a fork.

Snap the stem end off each green bean and then snap the beans into 1-inch sections. Add the green beans to the pot with the boiling potatoes during their last minute of cooking. This will take the raw edge off the beans, but still leave them slightly crisp.

Drain the potatoes and green beans in a colander. The heat from the potatoes will continue to cook the beans slightly as they drain.

In a large bowl, combine the green onions, mayonnaise, mustard, sugar, thyme, salt, and some black pepper and whisk until well combined. Taste the dressing and adjust the pepper, if needed.

Add the slightly cooled potatoes and green beans to the bowl with the dressing. Stir the salad to coat the potatoes and green beans in the dressing, slightly mashing the potatoes as you stir. Serve immediately or refrigerate until ready to eat.

 Chef's Tip: The flavor of the thyme will infuse into the salad as it refrigerates, making the flavor even better the next day!

Southwest Chicken Salad $$

Serves 4

I love chicken salad, but the price of chicken breasts can make it less than economical. Enter black beans and corn. Not only will these two ingredients stretch the salad and lower the cost per serving, but they also add flavor, texture, and nutrients. This chicken salad is so delicious that you'll want to eat it by itself, although I suggest stuffing it in a pita, eating it with crackers, or piling it over a bed of tender greens.

INGREDIENTS

1 pound boneless, skinless chicken breast

1 teaspoon chili powder

Pinch of salt

Pinch of freshly ground black pepper

1 (15-ounce) can black beans, drained and rinsed

2 to 3 green onions

½ bunch cilantro, roughly chopped

1 cup frozen corn kernels, thawed

¼ cup mayonnaise

¼ cup sour cream

1½ tablespoons apple cider vinegar

1 teaspoon ground cumin

¼ teaspoon salt

INSTRUCTIONS

Cut the chicken breast into 1-inch cubes and sprinkle with the chili powder, salt, and pepper.

Coat a medium skillet with nonstick cooking spray and add the chicken. Sauté the chicken over medium heat until it is no longer pink inside. Allow the chicken to cool and then roughly chop into small pieces.

In a large bowl, combine the beans, green onions, cilantro, and corn and toss to combine.

In a small bowl, combine the mayonnaise, sour cream, apple cider vinegar, cumin, and salt and stir until combined.

Add the chopped cooled chicken and dressing to the bowl. Stir until everything is combined and well coated in dressing. Cover and refrigerate until ready to serve.

 BUDGET BYTE To get the best price on chicken breasts, buy larger quantities or value packs, divide them into single portions, and then freeze them for later use.

Six

PASTA

Pasta is the poor man's best friend. It's quick, filling, extremely inexpensive, has a long shelf life, and is a completely blank canvas for flavor. With innovations in whole-wheat, low-carb, and gluten-free pasta, there's a pasta to fit just about anyone's dietary need. Keep your pantry stocked with shelf-stable dried pasta for quick, no-brainer dinners that can be spruced up with just a few flavorful ingredients. Here are a few ideas!

Spinach & Artichoke Pasta   *100*

Roasted Eggplant Pasta   *102*

Loaded Enchilada Pasta   *104*

Creamy Orzo with Spinach   *106*

Garlic-Herb Pasta   *108*

Pasta with Tuna & Olives   *109*

One-Skillet Lasagna   *111*

Easy Pad Thai   *112*

Sesame Noodles   *114*

Lemon-Parmesan Pasta with Peas   *115*

Zucchini-Pasta Bake   *116*

Spinach & Artichoke Pasta $$

Serves 6

I think we can all admit that at some point or another we've wanted to go to a restaurant and just order appetizers for dinner—especially the spinach and artichoke dip. Well, this pasta is a sneaky way to do just that. It's lighter than the average restaurant dip, but still has all the flavor and creamy goodness. Spinach and artichoke dip can be pricey, thanks to the artichokes and cheese, but adding pasta stretches the flavor, keeps the cost per serving in check, and turns it into a legit meal. Feel free to indulge!

INGREDIENTS

1 (10-ounce) package frozen chopped spinach, thawed

12 ounces bow-tie pasta

2 tablespoons olive oil

4 cloves garlic

¼ cup dry white wine

4 ounces Neufchâtel cheese

½ cup light sour cream

½ cup milk

½ cup grated Parmesan

1 (14-ounce) can quartered artichoke hearts

1 tablespoon hot sauce

Salt (optional)

Freshly ground black pepper (optional)

INSTRUCTIONS

Squeeze as much excess water from the spinach as possible. Set the spinach aside.

Bring a large pot of water to a rolling boil. Add the pasta and cook for 7 to 10 minutes, or until tender.

In a large skillet, heat the olive oil over medium heat. Add the garlic and sauté for 1 to 2 minutes, or just until it begins to soften. Add the wine, Neufchâtel, and sour cream and whisk the mixture until it is smooth and heated through. Reduce the heat to medium-low, then add the milk and Parmesan and whisk until the Parmesan has melted and the sauce is smooth.

Roughly chop the artichoke hearts into bite-size pieces and add them to the skillet along with the thawed spinach and hot sauce. Stir until well combined with the cream sauce. Taste and season with salt and pepper, if desired.

Drain the pasta well and add it to the skillet with the sauce. Stir to combine the pasta and sauce, then serve. If there is too much pasta to fit in the skillet, simply return the drained pasta to its cooking pot (with the heat turned off) and add the sauce to the pot. Stir to combine and then serve.

 BUDGET BYTE If you don't have any white wine on hand, substitute the same volume of chicken broth or more milk.

Roasted Eggplant Pasta $

Eggplant is highly underrated, but I think that's because most people don't know what to do with it. Raw eggplant can be bitter and has a texture similar to a sponge, but when it's roasted it becomes a rich and creamy delight. Combined with a simple tomato sauce and tangy feta cheese, this deceptively easy and elegant pasta has loads of flavor.

INGREDIENTS

1 large eggplant (about 1 pound), cut into 1-inch cubes

¼ cup olive oil

Pinch of salt

8 ounces linguine

2 cloves garlic, minced

1 (15-ounce) can diced tomatoes

½ teaspoon dried basil

¼ bunch fresh flat-leaf parsley, roughly chopped

2 ounces feta cheese, crumbled

INSTRUCTIONS

Preheat the oven to 400°F. Line a rimmed baking sheet with foil and then lightly coat the foil with nonstick cooking spray.

Spread the cubed eggplant out over the prepared baking sheet, drizzle it with 2 tablespoons of the olive oil, and toss to coat. Sprinkle the salt over the eggplant. Roast the eggplant for 30 minutes.

Bring a large pot of water to a rolling boil. Add the pasta to the boiling water and cook for 7 to 10 minutes, or until tender. Drain the pasta well and set aside.

In a skillet, heat the remaining 2 tablespoons olive oil over medium-low heat. Add the garlic and cook for 2 to 3 minutes, or until it is tender.

Add the diced tomatoes and their juices and the dried basil to the skillet and stir to combine. Stir the roasted eggplant into the tomato sauce. Add the drained pasta and stir again to combine. Remove the skillet from the heat.

Sprinkle the parsley and feta over the pasta and serve.

 Chef's Tip: Eggplant tends to soak up olive oil like a sponge, so it won't completely coat the outside of the cubes. The absorbed olive oil will still help the eggplant soften and prevent it from drying out, but you'll also need a thin layer of nonstick cooking spray to prevent the eggplant from sticking to the foil.

Loaded Enchilada Pasta

$

Serves 6

The last time I ate loaded nachos, I realized there was just no way to do it gracefully. My fingers got goopy, guacamole got on my face, and the toppings were constantly falling off the chips. It was a frustrating (albeit delicious) experience. So I started to think about ways to put all of those nacho toppings onto pasta so that I could eat it with a fork (and *hopefully* look good doing so). The key to making the idea work is my homemade Red Enchilada Sauce (page 77), which helps everything stick together in one easy-to-eat forkful after another. The creation of this Loaded Enchilada Pasta may be my proudest moment yet. Make it once and you'll see why.

INGREDIENTS

1 tablespoon vegetable oil

2 cloves garlic, minced

1 (10-ounce) can diced tomatoes with chiles (such as Rotel)

8 ounces wide egg noodles

1 (15-ounce) can black beans, drained and rinsed

½ cup frozen corn kernels

1 cup Red Enchilada Sauce (page 77; see Budget Byte, at right)

3 green onions, sliced

1 cup shredded cheddar

¼ bunch fresh cilantro, roughly chopped (optional)

INSTRUCTIONS

In a large skillet, heat the vegetable oil over medium-low heat. Add the garlic and sauté for 2 minutes, or until the garlic has softened slightly.

Add the diced tomatoes and their juices and 2 cups of water to the skillet and stir to combine. Add the uncooked egg noodles, cover the skillet, and raise the heat to medium-high.

Bring the mixture to a simmer, then reduce the heat to medium-low. Simmer for 10 minutes, stirring once halfway through, until the noodles have absorbed most of the liquid and become tender. The liquid in the skillet will not completely cover the uncooked noodles, but the steam trapped by the skillet's lid will help them cook.

Add the black beans, corn, and enchilada sauce to the skillet and stir to combine them with the noodles. Cook for about 5 minutes or until the black beans and corn are heated through.

Sprinkle the green onions over the pasta, followed by the cheese. Cover the skillet and allow the pasta to heat for a few more minutes, or until the cheese has melted. Sprinkle the cilantro over the pasta just before serving, if desired.

 BUDGET BYTE The enchilada sauce recipe yields 2 cups, but you can prepare a half batch by dividing the ingredient measures in half.

Creamy Orzo with Spinach $

Serves 6

This pasta dish reminds me of risotto, but requires only a fraction of the work. Light and tangy goat cheese melts right into the hot pasta and creates an instant cream sauce. Goat cheese is usually sold in small logs (sometimes labeled "chèvre") and can be found in the specialty cheese section. Although it can be relatively expensive, only a small amount is needed to add flavor and texture to this dish. Look for orzo, a small rice-shaped pasta, in the pasta aisle or bulk dry goods section.

INGREDIENTS

1 pound orzo

2 tablespoons salted butter

¼ teaspoon granulated garlic

¼ teaspoon red pepper flakes

¾ teaspoon salt

Freshly cracked black pepper

1 (10-ounce) package frozen chopped spinach, thawed

4 ounces goat cheese

INSTRUCTIONS

Bring a large pot of water to a rolling boil. Add the orzo and cook for 7 to 10 minutes, or until tender. Drain the orzo, reserving ½ cup of the starchy cooking water, and return the orzo to the pot with the heat turned off.

Add the butter, garlic, red pepper flakes, salt, and black pepper to the pasta. Stir to melt the butter and combine.

Squeeze as much moisture out of the thawed spinach as possible and add the spinach and goat cheese to the pasta. Stir to combine. The residual heat from the pasta will melt the goat cheese, creating a creamy coating over the pasta and spinach. If the mixture becomes dry or too sticky while stirring, add a small amount of the warm reserved pasta cooking water to loosen it up. Serve warm.

BUDGET BYTE For those on an extra-tight budget, or if goat cheese is unavailable in your area, try using 4 ounces of cream cheese instead. Cream cheese has a similar tang, but tends to be slightly thicker and heavier in texture than goat cheese.

Chef's Tip: Make sure to purchase frozen chopped spinach. Spinach that is frozen whole has a stringy texture and will not stir into the orzo well.

Garlic-Herb Pasta $

Serves 4   It's the little things in life. Simple flavors like garlic, butter, herbs, and Parmesan are all pasta needs to be heavenly. If you've ever made garlic-herb pasta from a packet mix and been underwhelmed, you might be surprised at how amazing it can *really* be when made fresh. It's quick, simple, delicious, and makes the perfect side to almost any meal.

INGREDIENTS

8 ounces pasta (any shape—angel hair and bow-tie are my favorite)

4 tablespoons salted butter

4 cloves garlic, minced

1 teaspoon dried basil

½ teaspoon salt

Freshly cracked black pepper

¼ bunch fresh flat-leaf parsley, roughly chopped

¼ cup grated Parmesan

INSTRUCTIONS

Bring a large pot of water to a rolling boil. Add the pasta and cook for 7 to 10 minutes, or until tender. Drain the pasta, reserving about ½ cup of the starchy pasta cooking water. Add the butter to the empty pasta pot and set the pot over medium-low heat to melt the butter. Add the garlic and sauté for 1 to 2 minutes, or just until the garlic begins to soften.

Return the cooked pasta to the pot, remove from the heat, and add the basil, salt, and black pepper to taste. Toss the pasta to coat it in the butter and seasoning. If the pasta becomes dry as you toss it, add a splash of the reserved pasta cooking water to help loosen it up. Add the chopped parsley and toss to combine with the pasta. Sprinkle the Parmesan over the top and serve.

Pasta with Tuna & Olives $$$

This pasta salad is insanely easy and packed with flavor, thanks to the kalamata olives, *Serves 8*
tuna, and Parmesan. Cherry tomatoes and a little fresh parsley help brighten and balance
the flavors. The dish is equally delicious warm or cold—on a hot summer night, a cold
bowl with a chilled glass of white wine is absolute heaven, and at a fraction of the price of
a restaurant meal. So, invite some friends over, make up a big batch of this pasta, and
enjoy life!

INGREDIENTS

1 pound bow-tie pasta

2 tablespoons olive oil

1 tablespoon red wine vinegar

½ teaspoon dried basil

Freshly cracked black pepper

1 pint cherry tomatoes, halved

2 (5-ounce) cans chunk light tuna in
water, drained

1 cup pitted kalamata olives, roughly
chopped

¼ bunch fresh flat-leaf parsley, roughly
chopped

¼ cup grated Parmesan

INSTRUCTIONS

Bring a large pot of water to a rolling boil. Add the pasta and cook for 7 to 10 minutes,
or until tender. Drain the pasta in a colander and set aside to cool slightly.

In a small bowl, whisk together the olive oil, vinegar, basil, and black pepper to taste.

Place the cherry tomatoes, tuna, olives, and parsley in a large bowl. Add the pasta, oil-
and-vinegar dressing, and Parmesan to the bowl and stir until well combined.

BUDGET BYTE Cherry tomatoes can be quite expensive, but can be substituted with chopped Roma tomatoes. They are usually less expensive, although they are not quite as sweet and do not look quite as nice as cherry tomatoes in the salad.

BUDGET BYTE It may be more economical to buy one larger can of tuna instead of two smaller cans, but be sure to check the price, as this is not always the case.

One-Skillet Lasagna $$

Serves 6

I *love* lasagna, but I *hate* all the time and prep work required to make it. This super-quick skillet version gives me all the flavor and ooey-gooey cheesy goodness without me spending hours in the kitchen. It may not be a pretty, layered casserole like a classic lasagna, but its rustic appearance has a charm of its own!

INGREDIENTS

2 tablespoons olive oil

2 cloves garlic, minced

½ pound Italian sausage (hot or sweet)

¼ cup tomato paste

1 (28-ounce) can diced tomatoes

1 teaspoon Italian seasoning blend

8 ounces wide egg noodles

¼ cup grated Parmesan

1 cup shredded mozzarella

INSTRUCTIONS

In a large skillet, heat the olive oil over medium heat. Add the garlic and cook for 1 to 2 minutes, or just until the garlic begins to soften. If the sausage is in a casing, remove and discard the casing. Add the sausage to the skillet and cook until thoroughly browned, breaking the sausage into small pieces with the side of a wooden spoon as it cooks. Drain the excess fat from the skillet.

Add the tomato paste, diced tomatoes, Italian seasoning, and 1½ cups of water to the skillet with the sausage. Stir the mixture, scraping any browned bits from the bottom of the skillet.

Add the pasta to the skillet and submerge it as much as possible under the sauce. Cover the skillet and allow the mixture to come to a simmer. Simmer, covered, stirring once or twice to prevent the pasta from sticking, for 15 minutes, or until the pasta is tender and has absorbed most of the liquid. Sprinkle the Parmesan over the pasta, followed by the mozzarella. Cover and cook for 5 minutes more, or until the cheese has melted. Serve hot.

Easy Pad Thai $$

I'm probably not supposed to play favorites, but this recipe is *definitely* my favorite. Pad thai is the epitome of simple ingredients creating dazzling flavor. It's fresh, light, exotic, and faster than any takeout (unless, of course, you happen to live above a restaurant that delivers). Fresh lime is key to creating the unique flavor, but one lime should be enough for a single or even double batch of this noodle dish. Fish sauce, which you can find in the Asian section of most major grocery stores or at Asian markets, gives this pasta a more authentic flavor, but if you can't find any, skip it; this dish will still rock your world.

INGREDIENTS

8 ounces pad thai or lo mein noodles

2 tablespoons vegetable oil

1 clove garlic, minced

2 large eggs

1½ tablespoons soy sauce

2 tablespoons fresh lime juice (from about 1 medium lime)

2 tablespoons brown sugar

1 teaspoon fish sauce

⅛ teaspoon red pepper flakes

3 green onions, sliced

¼ bunch fresh cilantro, leaves only, roughly chopped

¼ cup chopped, unsalted peanuts

INSTRUCTIONS

Bring a large pot of water to a rolling boil. Add the noodles and cook for 7 to 10 minutes, or until tender. Drain the noodles and set aside.

In a large skillet, heat the vegetable oil over medium heat. Add the garlic and cook for 1 to 2 minutes, or until tender.

Whisk the eggs lightly with a fork. Pour them into the skillet and cook just until they solidify, but are still moist, moving the eggs around the skillet slightly as they cook so that they lightly scramble. When the eggs are cooked, remove the skillet from the heat and set aside.

In a small bowl, stir together the soy sauce, lime juice, sugar, fish sauce, and red pepper flakes. Pour the sauce into the skillet with the scrambled eggs. Add the noodles and toss to coat in the sauce.

Sprinkle the green onions, cilantro, and peanuts over the noodles. Toss lightly to combine. Serve warm.

 BUDGET BYTE Pad thai noodles have a unique flavor and texture, but if you can't find them in your area, try substituting another flat pasta like linguine.

 Chef's Tip: To get the most juice from your lime, roll it on your countertop while applying pressure before cutting it open. This causes the juice capsules to burst and release more juice.

Sesame Noodles

Serves 4

Warning: This pasta is *really* addictive (as if pasta needs any help in that area, right?). This super-simple Asian sauce tickles all of your taste buds with elements of sweet, salty, and spicy, and a smooth, nutty richness. You can serve this as a side to other Asian-inspired dishes, like Teriyaki Salmon with Sriracha Mayo (page 173), or as a bed under stir-fried vegetables, chicken, or tofu.

INGREDIENTS

8 ounces angel hair pasta

3 tablespoons salted butter

3 cloves garlic, minced

3 tablespoons soy sauce

3 tablespoons rice vinegar

3 tablespoons brown sugar

½ teaspoon toasted sesame oil

⅛ teaspoon red pepper flakes

2 tablespoons tahini (sesame seed paste)

2 green onions, sliced

INSTRUCTIONS

Bring a large pot of water to a rolling boil. Add the pasta and cook for 7 to 10 minutes, or until tender. Drain the pasta and set aside.

In a large skillet, melt the butter over medium-low heat. Add the garlic and sauté for 2 minutes, or just until the garlic begins to soften.

In a small bowl, stir together the soy sauce, vinegar, sugar, sesame oil, and red pepper flakes.

Add the cooked pasta to the skillet, pour the sauce over the top, and toss to coat. Stir the tahini into the pasta mixture, toss to coat, and allow the residual heat to melt the tahini into the sauce. Sprinkle the green onions over the top and serve.

Lemon-Parmesan Pasta with Peas $

Serves 4

This pasta has spring written all over it. The bright flavor of lemon and the sweetness of green peas create a light, fresh flavor. It can be served warm or cold, making it perfect for picnics, potlucks, or just a weeknight dinner on the patio. Sometimes the fewer ingredients you have, the more their flavor can shine through.

INGREDIENTS

8 ounces orecchiette or shell-shaped pasta

1 cup frozen sweet peas

1 medium lemon

2 tablespoons salted butter

Salt

Freshly cracked black pepper

¼ cup grated Parmesan

INSTRUCTIONS

Bring a large pot of water to a boil. Add the pasta and cook for 7 to 10 minutes, or until tender. Add the frozen peas to the boiling pasta during the last minute of cooking to quickly blanch them. Drain the pasta and peas in a colander and set aside.

Using a Microplane or a small-holed cheese grater, scrape off the thin, yellow layer of zest from the lemon (do not grate down to the white pith). Juice the lemon into a small bowl and set aside.

In a large skillet, melt the butter over medium-low heat. Add the lemon zest and simmer it in the butter for 1 to 2 minutes.

Add the drained pasta and peas to the skillet and toss to coat in the lemon butter. Add the reserved lemon juice and season with salt and pepper to taste. Remove the pan from the heat.

Sprinkle the pasta with the Parmesan and toss to coat.

Zucchini-Pasta Bake

Serves 6

Some kind of magic happens when zucchini is cooked: It develops this amazingly rich, almost buttery flavor that I can't get enough of. I could happily eat bowls of sautéed zucchini by itself, but when I decided to combine it with pasta, marinara sauce, and a little mozzarella, I hit the jackpot. It was quick, easy, and left me satisfied without feeling weighed down. It's a fast, easy, and very welcome light alternative to traditional lasagna.

INGREDIENTS

12 ounces bow-tie pasta

1 medium zucchini

1 tablespoon olive oil

1 clove garlic, minced

1 teaspoon dried oregano

⅛ teaspoon salt

Freshly cracked black pepper

2 cups marinara sauce

¼ cup grated Parmesan

2 cups shredded mozzarella

INSTRUCTIONS

Preheat the oven to 350°F. Coat an 8-by-8-inch casserole dish with nonstick cooking spray.

Bring a large pot of water to a rolling boil. Add the pasta and cook for 7 to 10 minutes, or until tender. Drain the pasta in a colander and then return it to the pot with the heat turned off.

Slice the zucchini into ¼-inch-thick half-rounds. Add the olive oil, garlic, and zucchini to a medium skillet. Sprinkle the dried oregano, salt, and black pepper over the top. Sauté the zucchini over medium heat for about 5 minutes, or just until tender but not mushy. Transfer the sautéed zucchini to the pot with the pasta and add the marinara sauce. Stir until everything is coated in sauce. Add the Parmesan and 1 cup of the mozzarella. Stir until combined.

Pour the pasta into the prepared casserole dish. Sprinkle the remaining 1 cup mozzarella over the pasta. Bake for 30 minutes, or until heated through and bubbly.

 BUDGET BYTE After baking, divide the pasta into single-serving portions, allow it to cool in the refrigerator, and then freeze the pasta for quick, reheatable meals.

 BUDGET BYTE Shredded cheese freezes very well. To save money, buy large bags, divide them into 2-cup portions, and freeze them for later use. The frozen cheese thaws quickly at room temperature or in the refrigerator.

Seven

SOUPS

Soup has unfairly earned a bad reputation for being thin, watery, and unsatisfying. Sure, if you get your soup from a can, all of the above are probably true. Homemade soup, on the other hand, is anything but. Hearty, warm, filling, and bursting with flavor—that's what homemade soup is all about. Even better, soup is usually a quick fix, rarely requires more than one pot or pan, and almost always freezes well. Keep your freezer stocked with a variety of soups for those cold nights when you need something warm to soothe your soul.

Chinese Chicken Noodle Soup *120*

Tomato-Cheddar Soup *122*

Carrot–Sweet Potato Soup *124*

Lentil & Sausage Stew *126*

Pasta e Fagioli *128*

Curried Potato & Pea Soup *130*

Broccoli & Cheddar Soup *132*

Better-Than-Mom's Chili *134*

Hearty Vegetable & Barley Soup *136*

Greek Lemon & Orzo Soup *138*

Zesty Black Bean Soup *139*

Chinese Chicken Noodle Soup $$

Serves 8

Homemade chicken noodle soup is always warm and comforting, but when you add fresh ginger and Chinese five-spice powder, an intoxicating blend of cinnamon, black pepper, ginger, fennel, and anise, you create an ultra-aromatic soup that will soothe the body, mind, and soul. I like to keep single-serving portions of this soup in my freezer for days when I'm feeling under the weather, am too tired to cook, or just need a hot bowl of something comforting. This exotic twist on a home-cooked classic is sure to become a family favorite.

INGREDIENTS

2 tablespoons vegetable oil

1 medium yellow onion, diced

2 cloves garlic, minced

4-inch piece fresh ginger, peeled

8 ounces button mushrooms, rinsed and sliced

1 boneless, skinless chicken breast (about ¾ pound)

4 cups chicken broth

2 tablespoons soy sauce

2 tablespoons rice vinegar

1 teaspoon Chinese five-spice powder

1 (3-ounce) package ramen noodles (seasoning discarded)

½ bunch green onions, sliced

INSTRUCTIONS

In a large pot, heat the vegetable oil over medium-low heat. Add the onion and garlic, and grate the ginger straight into the pot using a cheese grater or a Microplane. Sauté the onion, garlic, and ginger for about 5 minutes, or until the onion begins to soften.

Add the mushrooms, chicken breast, chicken broth, soy sauce, rice vinegar, five-spice powder, and 4 cups of water to the pot. Cover the pot, raise the heat to high, and allow the soup to come to a full boil. Reduce the heat to low and simmer, covered, for 30 minutes.

Carefully remove the chicken breast and use two forks to shred the meat. Return the shredded meat to the pot. Break the block of dry ramen noodles into a few pieces, add them to the soup, and continue simmering until the noodles are tender, about 5 minutes.

Add the green onions to the soup just before serving.

Chef's Tip: This soup is excellent for using up extra vegetables. I like to toss in extra baby spinach if I have it on hand, chop up a carrot or two, or even toss in a few broccoli florets.

You can buy packages of plain ramen noodles (without seasoning) at Asian markets or in the Asian section of your grocery store, but although they may be a slightly better quality, they are often much more expensive than that old college standby.

Tomato-Cheddar Soup

$

Serves 6

If regular tomato soup seems thin to you, you've got to try this thick, rich, and savory homemade version. It doesn't take much more work than heating up a can of premade soup, but it will taste like you've ordered out from the corner bistro. Throw a few chunky croutons on top and you won't even need a grilled cheese on the side.

INGREDIENTS

1 tablespoon olive oil

1 clove garlic, minced

½ small onion, diced

1 (28-ounce) can crushed tomatoes

3 cups chicken broth

¼ cup plain bread crumbs

1 teaspoon dried basil

½ tablespoon brown sugar

½ teaspoon salt, plus more as needed

Freshly cracked black pepper

1 cup shredded cheddar

INSTRUCTIONS

In a large pot, heat the olive oil over medium heat. Add the garlic and onion and cook for about 5 minutes, or until the onion has softened.

Add the crushed tomatoes, chicken broth, bread crumbs, basil, brown sugar, salt, and some pepper and stir to combine. Bring the mixture to a simmer and cook for 15 minutes.

Remove the pot from the heat and begin adding the cheese, a small amount at a time, whisking each addition until it is fully melted and incorporated before adding more. Taste the soup and adjust the salt and pepper as needed. Serve hot.

Chef's Tip: For an extra-smooth soup, use an immersion blender to puree the soup until smooth just before adding the cheese.

 Chef's Tip: For a vegetarian version, substitute vegetable broth for the chicken broth.

Carrot-Sweet Potato Soup

*Serves
6 to 8*

This beautifully vibrant and aromatic soup is deceptively easy to prepare, full of flavor, and low in calories. Cinnamon and allspice create a uniquely sweet and savory flavor that will transport you to exotic foreign lands. It's perfect for dipping chunks of crusty French bread or even sopping up with homemade Naan (page 56). Try adding a dollop of Greek yogurt for added creaminess or a splash of sriracha for a spicy kick.

INGREDIENTS

2 tablespoons olive oil

1 medium yellow onion, diced

2 cloves garlic, minced

2-inch piece fresh ginger, peeled

1 pound carrots, sliced crosswise into
½-inch rounds

1 medium sweet potato (1 to 1½ pounds),
peeled and cut into ½-inch cubes

6 cups chicken broth

1 teaspoon ground cinnamon

½ teaspoon ground allspice

½ teaspoon salt

Freshly cracked black pepper

INSTRUCTIONS

In a large pot, heat the olive oil over medium-low heat. Add the onion and garlic and grate the ginger directly into the pot using a small-holed cheese grater or a Microplane. Sauté for about 5 minutes, or until the onion begins to soften.

Add the carrots, sweet potato, chicken broth, cinnamon, and allspice to the pot and stir to combine. Cover the pot and raise the heat to high. Bring the soup to a boil, then reduce the heat to low. Let simmer, covered, for 15 minutes, or until the sweet potato and carrots are tender.

Using an immersion blender, puree the soup until smooth. Add the salt and pepper to taste. (Alternatively, if you do not have an immersion blender, allow the soup to cool until lukewarm, transfer it to a standing blender, and puree until smooth. Never blend hot soup or liquid as it can be very dangerous and cause severe burns.)

 Chef's Tip: Simply swapping vegetable broth for chicken broth makes this recipe vegan!

Lentil & Sausage Stew $

Serves
8 to 10

My first thought after tasting this recipe was, *Where have you been all my life?* and I've had several readers express the same. With the lentils, sausage, and mélange of vegetables, this stew is truly a meal in a bowl. Even better yet, it makes excellent leftovers. It is *so* good that I found myself doing a happy dance when I found a bowl of it in my freezer a few weeks later. I almost couldn't wait to reheat it and chow down. The earthy blend of spices only gets better after day one, so you'll definitely be scraping the bottom of the pot on this one.

INGREDIENTS

1 tablespoon olive oil

1 pound sweet Italian sausage, casings removed

½ pound carrots (about 3 medium), halved lengthwise and cut into half-moons

4 stalks celery, diced

1 medium onion, diced

2 cloves garlic, minced

2 cups brown lentils

6 cups chicken broth

1 teaspoon dried oregano

1 teaspoon ground cumin

1 teaspoon paprika

¼ teaspoon cayenne pepper

1 (10-ounce) package frozen spinach

INSTRUCTIONS

In a large soup pot, heat the olive oil over medium heat. Add the sausage and cook, breaking it up with the side of a wooden spoon, until browned, 5 to 7 minutes.

Add the carrots, celery, onion, and garlic to the pot and sauté for about 5 minutes, or until the onion has softened and become translucent.

Spread the lentils out on a baking sheet and pick out any small stones or debris. Rinse the lentils briefly in a colander and then add them to the pot along with the broth, oregano, cumin, paprika, and cayenne pepper.

Raise the heat to medium-high and bring the soup to a simmer. Simmer for 30 minutes, or until the lentils are tender. (Use a large spoon to retrieve a few lentils and test them for tenderness. They should not be hard in the center.)

Add the spinach to the soup (no thawing necessary) and simmer until thawed and heated through. Once the spinach is fully incorporated into the soup, taste and adjust the seasonings, if needed, and serve.

 Chef's Tip: Brown or green lentils will work for this recipe, although green lentils will require about 45 minutes of simmering, rather than 30 minutes, to soften. Red, orange, and yellow lentils lose their shape and become mushy when cooked, making them not well suited for this stew.

Pasta e Fagioli

$

Italians sure know how to do it right. This soup is insanely simple and it follows my Budget Byting formula to a tee. The soup relies on bulky, inexpensive ingredients, like pasta and beans, to fill you up, while just a small amount of bacon infuses the whole pot with intense flavor. Despite its extreme simplicity, this is one soup that keeps me coming back for seconds, and my freezer is stocked with this Pasta e Fagioli year-round.

INGREDIENTS

3 ounces bacon (3 to 4 slices), cut crosswise into ½-inch pieces

1 medium yellow onion

2 cloves garlic

1 (15-ounce) can diced tomatoes

1 (15-ounce) can white beans (Great Northern, navy, or cannellini), drained and rinsed

4 cups chicken broth

½ teaspoon dried oregano

½ teaspoon dried basil

1 cup ditalini (small, tube-shaped pasta)

¼ bunch fresh flat-leaf parsley, leaves only, roughly chopped

¼ cup grated Parmesan

INSTRUCTIONS

In a large pot, cook the bacon over medium heat for 7 to 10 minutes, or until it is crispy and most of the fat has rendered. (As the bacon browns, it may begin to stick to the bottom of the pot, but don't worry—it will dissolve into the soup later and provide big flavor.)

Add the onion and garlic to the pot and cook for about 5 minutes, or until the onion has softened.

Add the tomatoes and their juices to the pot. Stir well and scrape up any browned bits from the bottom of the pot.

Add the beans to the pot along with the chicken broth, oregano, and basil. Stir to combine. Cover the pot, raise the heat to high, and bring the soup to a boil.

Add the pasta to the boiling soup and stir to combine. Reduce the heat to low and simmer for 10 to 15 minutes, or until the pasta is fully cooked. Stir the fresh parsley into the soup and serve hot with a light sprinkling of Parmesan over each bowl.

 BUDGET BYTE I frequently use small amounts of bacon in recipes to add big flavor. Rather than freezing or using individual slices, I cut the package across the slices into four 3-ounce sections prior to freezing. That way, I can grab just the amount I need from the freezer and add it straight to the skillet.

 Chef's Tip: Cooking bacon can be intimidating, but don't be tempted to use precooked bacon instead. The fat that renders from the bacon while it cooks eliminates the need for extra cooking oil and is pivotal to achieving big flavor in the finished soup. Cooking bacon in the bottom of a large soup pot is much easier because the tall side walls minimize dangerous splattering of the hot rendered fat.

Curried Potato & Pea Soup

Serves 4 to 6

Potato soup is a classic, but I like to give it an exotic twist by adding curry powder. Blending the cooked potatoes into the soup creates a luxurious, velvety texture that balances the heady curry spices. A few sweet peas give the soup a touch of freshness, and suddenly you've got a fancy soup fit for a white linen napkin restaurant, at a fraction of the price. You can use either hot or mild curry powder, or adjust the heat yourself with a pinch or two of cayenne pepper. Garnish with a dollop of plain Greek yogurt, a few croutons, or even some dried pumpkin seeds.

INGREDIENTS

1 tablespoon olive oil

1 small yellow onion, diced

1 clove garlic, minced

1 pound russet potatoes, cut into
   1-inch cubes

4 cups chicken broth

½ tablespoon hot or mild curry powder,
   plus more as needed

1 cup frozen peas

INSTRUCTIONS

In a 4-quart saucepan, heat the olive oil over medium heat. Add the onion and garlic and cook for about 5 minutes, or until the onion has softened.

Add the potatoes, chicken broth, and curry powder and stir to combine. Cover the pot, raise the heat to high, and bring the mixture to a boil. Reduce the heat to low and simmer for about 10 minutes, or until the potatoes are very tender.

Using an immersion blender, puree the soup until smooth. (Alternatively, if you do not have an immersion blender, allow the soup to cool until lukewarm, transfer it to a standing blender, and puree until smooth. Never blend hot soup or liquid as it can be very dangerous and cause severe burns.)

Taste the soup and adjust the curry powder to your liking. Add the peas and cook until heated through, about 5 minutes. Serve hot.

 BUDGET BYTE Curry powder can be found in the spice aisle or ethnic foods aisle at most grocery stores, but you'll find the best prices at ethnic markets.

Broccoli & Cheddar Soup $$

Serves 6

Broccoli and cheddar soup—totally sinful, right? Well, it doesn't have to be. I make a lighter soup base that is still rich and creamy with a great cheddar flavor, but won't assault your arteries. In addition to lots of delicious broccoli, I like to add a little shredded carrot for a bright pop of color, extra texture, and a hint of natural sweetness. Served with a hearty roll, like my Multigrain Rolls (page 54), this makes for a warm and filling meal on a cold autumn night.

INGREDIENTS

1 broccoli crown (about ¾ pound)

2 medium carrots, grated

2 cups chicken broth

4 tablespoons salted butter

1 medium yellow onion, diced

2 cloves garlic, minced

¼ cup all-purpose flour

3 cups milk

¼ teaspoon ground nutmeg

8 ounces medium or sharp cheddar, shredded

¼ teaspoon salt

Freshly cracked black pepper

INSTRUCTIONS

Chop the broccoli, including the stems, into very small pieces. Combine the chopped broccoli, grated carrots, and chicken broth in a medium pot and bring to a boil over high heat. Cook for 3 to 5 minutes, or just until the broccoli is tender. Remove from the heat and set aside.

In a separate pot, melt the butter over medium-low heat. Add the onion and garlic and sauté for about 5 minutes, or until the onion is tender.

Add the flour to the pot with the onion mixture and whisk to combine. Continue to cook, stirring continually, for 2 minutes.

Warm the milk slightly in the microwave and then slowly whisk it into the pot with the onion-flour mixture. Once all the milk has been added, raise the heat to medium and allow the mixture to come to a gentle simmer, at which point it will begin to thicken. Stir in the nutmeg.

Slowly whisk the cheese, a handful at a time, into the sauce, whisking each addition until it is fully melted and incorporated before adding more. Stir in the cooked vegetables and broth. Add the salt, then taste the soup and add pepper as desired.

 BUDGET BYTE Substitute one 10-ounce package of frozen, chopped broccoli if fresh broccoli is expensive or unavailable in your area.

Better-Than-Mom's Chili

Serves 6 to 8

My mom's chili was one of my favorite meals growing up. I'll never forget the smell of ground beef and chili spices filling up our kitchen as the pot simmered on the stove. Her secret was using V8 juice as a base for the sauce, which gives it a rich, complex flavor.

I've been making her version for years, but recently have started experimenting and adding a few secret ingredients of my own. Smoked paprika, one of my new favorite spices, provides a subtle smoky mystique, and adding just a little bit of cocoa powder makes the sauce extra rich, thick, and earthy. I never thought I'd say it, but this chili is better than Mom's (sorry, Mom!).

INGREDIENTS

1 tablespoon olive oil

1 medium onion, diced

4 cloves garlic, minced

1 pound ground beef

1 (15-ounce) can diced tomatoes

1 (15-ounce) can kidney beans, drained and rinsed

1 (15-ounce) can pinto beans, drained and rinsed

1 (15-ounce) can black beans, drained and rinsed

3 cups vegetable juice blend (such as V8)

1 tablespoon chili powder

1 teaspoon ground cumin

½ teaspoon dried oregano

¼ teaspoon cayenne pepper

1 teaspoon smoked paprika

1½ tablespoons unsweetened cocoa powder

½ tablespoon brown sugar

1 teaspoon salt, plus more as needed

INSTRUCTIONS

In a large soup pot, heat the olive oil over medium-low heat. Add the onion and garlic and sauté for about 5 minutes, or until the onion is soft and translucent.

Add the ground beef and sauté until it is fully browned. Add the diced tomatoes and their juices, the kidney, pinto, and black beans, and the vegetable juice blend, chili powder, cumin, oregano, cayenne, smoked paprika, cocoa powder, and brown sugar. Stir to combine.

Raise the heat to medium-high and bring the mixture to a simmer. Simmer, uncovered, for about 15 minutes. Add the salt; taste the chili and adjust the seasoning with more salt, if desired. Serve hot.

Chef's Tip: You may smell a burst of chocolate when you add the cocoa powder to the chili, but the flavor soon blends in and creates a deep richness that is hard to put your finger on. Don't worry—your finished chili will not taste like a chocolate bar.

BUDGET BYTE Most large grocery stores carry generic (cheaper) brands of vegetable juice. Thirty-two-ounce cans are often much less expensive than their 32-ounce plastic bottle counterparts, but they are not resealable. Leftover vegetable juice can be frozen for use in other recipes or for a delicious Bloody Mary for your weekend brunch.

Hearty Vegetable & Barley Soup $

Serves 8

This might just be my new favorite soup. It's super filling, has a *ton* of vegetables, and doesn't require any bouillon or premade broth. The medley of delicious vegetables creates its own amazingly flavorful broth and a little pearled barley adds just enough *oomph* to make it soup-er filling (I couldn't resist). This recipe makes a large pot, but it freezes extremely well, so save some for a rainy day!

INGREDIENTS

2 tablespoons olive oil

2 cloves garlic, minced

1 medium onion, diced

2 medium carrots, sliced crosswise into rounds

2 stalks celery, diced

1 large potato, cut into ½-inch cubes

1 (28-ounce) can diced tomatoes

½ cup frozen peas

½ cup pearled barley

1 teaspoon dried oregano

1 teaspoon dried basil

1 bay leaf

Freshly cracked black pepper

1½ teaspoons salt

INGREDIENTS

In a large pot, heat the olive oil over medium-low heat. Add the garlic and onion and cook for about 5 minutes, or until the onion has softened.

Add the carrot, celery, and potato to the pot and continue to sauté for 2 to 3 minutes more.

Add the diced tomatoes and their juices, the peas, barley, oregano, basil, bay leaf, about 10 to 15 cranks of pepper, and 3 cups of water. Stir to combine. Cover the pot, raise the heat to high, and allow the mixture to come to a boil. Reduce the heat to low and simmer for 30 minutes, or until the barley is tender.

Once the barley is tender, add the salt. Taste the soup and adjust seasoning as needed. Remove and discard the bay leaf, and serve hot.

 BUDGET BYTE Buying pearled barley from bulk bins is often less expensive than buying prepackaged barley, plus you can buy any amount you need. Uncooked barley is great to have on hand, since it has an indefinite shelf life when stored in an airtight container away from heat and moisture.

Greek Lemon & Orzo Soup $

Serves 4

This soup is super quick and packed with fresh flavor. It makes an excellent side to a half sandwich, or a light lunch on its own. The bright, lemony broth is made mellow and creamy by the surprising addition of an egg. You can add more to this simple soup by stirring in some fresh spinach or even a cup or two of shredded rotisserie chicken.

INGREDIENTS

1 tablespoon olive oil

1 small onion, diced

1 clove garlic, minced

1 medium lemon

3 cups chicken broth

½ cup orzo

1 large egg

¼ bunch fresh flat-leaf parsley, roughly chopped

INSTRUCTIONS

In a large pot, heat the olive oil over medium-low heat. Add the onion and garlic and sauté for about 5 minutes, or until the onions have softened. Using a Microplane or a small-holed cheese grater, scrape off the thin yellow layer of zest from the lemon (do not grate down to the white pith). Stir the lemon zest into the onion mixture. Reserve the lemon.

Add the chicken broth and 1 cup of water to the pot. Raise the heat to high and bring the mixture to a boil. Add the orzo, reduce the heat to medium, and simmer for about 10 minutes, or until the orzo is tender. Remove the pot from the heat.

Juice the reserved lemon into a small bowl. In a medium bowl, whisk together the egg and lemon juice. Slowly whisk about ½ cup of the hot soup into the egg mixture to temper the eggs (this will prevent the eggs from curdling or "scrambling" in the hot liquid). Whisking constantly, pour the egg mixture back into the pot with the remaining hot soup. The soup should have a thick, almost creamy consistency.

Stir the parsley into the soup just before serving. Serve hot.

Zesty Black Bean Soup

Serves 4 to 6

I remember watching a guy I had a crush on in college make a pot of black bean soup and thinking, *Wow, this guy really knows how to cook!* Well, ladies and gentlemen, now that I'm much older and wiser, I no longer fall for such parlor tricks. Black bean soup is one of the easiest and most flavorful soups around. Earthy black beans and smoky cumin are such a great flavor combination that you barely need to add anything else to make a spectacular soup. I've added a few more ingredients, like carrot and jalapeño, to make it a bit more interesting, but this soup is simplicity at its best. So, whether you want a delicious, hearty bowl of soup for yourself, or you're just trying to make it *look* like you know what you're doing, this soup will get the job done.

INGREDIENTS

2 tablespoons olive oil

1 small yellow onion, diced

4 cloves garlic, minced

1 small jalapeño, seeded and diced

1 medium carrot, shredded

2 (15-ounce) cans black beans

1 (15-ounce) can diced tomatoes

2 cups chicken broth

1 teaspoon ground cumin

2 bay leaves

¼ teaspoon salt

INSTRUCTIONS

In a large pot, heat the olive oil over medium-low heat. Add the onion and garlic and sauté for about 5 minutes, or until the onions have softened.

Add the jalapeño and carrot to the pot and sauté the vegetables for 2 to 3 minutes more.

Add the black beans and their liquid as well as the diced tomatoes and their juices to the pot. Stir to combine. Add the chicken broth, cumin, and bay leaves, cover the pot, and bring the mixture to a simmer. Simmer for 15 minutes, then remove and discard the bay leaves.

Using an immersion blender, puree the soup until smooth. (Alternatively, if you do not have an immersion blender, allow the soup to cool until lukewarm, transfer it to a standing blender, and puree until smooth. Never blend hot soup or liquid as it can be very dangerous and cause severe burns.)

Season with the salt and serve hot.

 Chef's Tip: Always be careful when blending hot soups. Allow the soup to cool to the point where it will no longer burn the skin on contact, and place a dishtowel over the lid of the blender to catch any possible spray or splatter.

I t's true, I eat vegetarian more often than not. After all, it's economical, and with such a great variety of fresh fruits, vegetables, and grains, I never get bored. That being said, I *really* enjoy the occasional hearty piece of meat! Meat *can* be consumed on a budget, but you've got to be smart about it; buy meat when it's on sale and freeze it for later use; use sensible portions; and always bulk out your meal with inexpensive items like beans, grains, and vegetables.

Farmer Joes *142*

Ginger Beef 'n' Broccoli *144*

Chili-Cheese Beef 'n' Mac *146*

Greek Steak Tacos *148*

Beef & Bean Taquitos *150*

Spicy Beef 'n' Noodles *152*

Coconut Chicken Curry *154*

Turkey Florentine Meatballs *156*

Chicken Tamale Pie *158*

Rosemary-Garlic Roasted Chicken & Potatoes *160*

Teriyaki Chicken Sliders *162*

Chorizo–Sweet Potato Enchiladas *164*

Five-Spice Chops *166*

Herb-Roasted Pork Loin *167*

Pork with Balsamic-Cranberry Sauce *169*

Asian Pork Lettuce Wraps *171*

Teriyaki Salmon with Sriracha Mayo *173*

Lemon-Garlic Shrimp Pasta *175*

Thai Steamed Fish *177*

Farmer Joes $$

Serves 6

Sloppy Joes are delicious, but they don't really make a well-rounded meal. Beef, bread, and a sugary sauce don't exactly hit all the nutritional bases, so I like to make Farmer Joes instead. I cut the beef in half and bulk out the recipe with vegetables, which not only lowers the cost, but also enhances the flavor, texture, and nutritional content. This recipe is a total winner for your taste buds, wallet, and body. Oh, and don't be intimidated by the long ingredient list; the recipe whips up surprisingly fast and with minimal effort.

INGREDIENTS

2 tablespoons vegetable oil

1 medium yellow onion, diced

2 cloves garlic, minced

1 medium bell pepper, seeded and diced

2 medium carrots, grated

1 small zucchini, grated

½ pound lean ground beef

1 cup frozen corn kernels

1 (15-ounce) can diced tomatoes

1 (6-ounce) can tomato paste

3 tablespoons apple cider vinegar

2 tablespoons brown sugar

1 tablespoon Dijon mustard

1 teaspoon chili powder

1½ teaspoons salt

6 whole-wheat buns or pita pockets

INSTRUCTIONS

In a large skillet, heat the vegetable oil over medium-low heat. Add the onion and garlic and sauté for about 5 minutes, or until the onions have softened.

Add the bell pepper to the skillet and continue to sauté. Add the carrot and zucchini and stir to combine. Raise the heat to medium and sauté for about 10 minutes, or until most of the moisture on the bottom of the skillet has evaporated.

Add the ground beef and cook until the beef is completely browned, 5 to 7 minutes. Stir in the frozen corn kernels.

Add the diced tomatoes and their juices, the tomato paste, vinegar, brown sugar, mustard, chili powder, and salt and stir to combine. Continue to cook for about 10 minutes, or until heated through. Serve on whole-wheat buns or stuffed into pita pockets.

 BUDGET BYTE This is one of my favorite dishes to freeze. I freeze the beef filling in single-serving portions, which I can then quickly reheat in the microwave or a saucepan for an almost instant weeknight dinner.

Ginger Beef 'n' Broccoli

$$ \$\$ $$

Serves 4

Recipes like this are staples at Chinese-American fast-food restaurants for two reasons: They're fast, and they're delicious. By whipping up this dish at home, you'll be in complete control over the ingredient quality and sodium content. Beef can be quite expensive, especially in steak form, but when you bulk it up with fresh broccoli and jasmine rice, the price per serving becomes quite affordable.

INGREDIENTS

1 clove garlic, minced

3-inch piece fresh ginger, peeled and grated

2 tablespoons vegetable oil

1 tablespoon soy sauce

½ tablespoon rice vinegar

½ pound sirloin tip steak, cut across the grain into ⅛-inch-thick strips

1 head broccoli, chopped into bite-size florets

2 tablespoons oyster sauce

1 tablespoon cornstarch

4 cups cooked jasmine rice, warm

INSTRUCTIONS

Place the garlic, ginger, vegetable oil, soy sauce, and vinegar in a quart-size zip-top bag.

Place the sliced steak in the bag with the marinade and toss briefly to coat. Place the bag in the refrigerator and allow the steak to marinate for at least 30 minutes.

Bring a large pot of water to a boil over high heat. Add the broccoli and cook for 2 minutes, or just until it is tender-crisp. Drain the broccoli in a colander and then rinse it briefly with cool water to stop the cooking process.

Heat a large skillet over medium-high heat. Add the beef and all of the marinade to the hot skillet. Sauté the mixture until the beef is cooked through, 5 to 7 minutes.

In a small dish, combine the oyster sauce, cornstarch, and ½ cup of water and stir until well mixed. Pour the mixture over the beef. Allow the sauce to come to a simmer and thicken.

Add the cooked broccoli to the skillet and toss to coat it in the sauce. Serve the beef and broccoli over the warm jasmine rice.

Chef's Tip: For faster prep, you can substitute frozen florets for the fresh broccoli. The frozen broccoli is already partially cooked and does not need to be parboiled before it is added to the sauce.

BUDGET BYTE To freeze this dish, spoon the rice and beef mixture into individual, single-serving, resealable, freezer-safe containers. To reheat, simply microwave until warmed through.

Chili-Cheese Beef 'n' Mac

$$ \$\$ $$

Serves 6

I love trying to re-create boxed "skillet meals" at home. The preparation method is usually the same, but I'm in control of the ingredients. The only convenience lost is having everything premeasured, which, let's face it, only takes a few minutes. This recipe is my version of those classic Hamburger Helper meals from your childhood. It's fast, hearty, cheesy, and comforting. If you are new to cooking and not quite ready to experiment with ethnic flavors, this recipe is the perfect place to start. Its familiar flavor has everything you already know you love: pasta, beef, tomato, and cheese.

INGREDIENTS

1 tablespoon olive oil

1 pound lean ground beef

2 cloves garlic, minced

1 small onion, diced

2 tablespoons all-purpose flour

2 cups beef broth (see Budget Byte, at right)

1 (8-ounce) can tomato sauce

1 tablespoon chili powder

½ teaspoon smoked paprika (optional)

½ teaspoon dried oregano

2 cups elbow macaroni

1 cup (4 ounces) shredded sharp cheddar

INSTRUCTIONS

In a large pot, heat the olive oil over medium heat. Add the ground beef and cook until the beef is fully browned, 5 to 7 minutes.

Add the garlic and onion to the beef and continue to sauté for 5 minutes, or until the onion is soft and translucent. Add the flour and cook, stirring, for 1 minute more. (It's okay if the flour begins to coat the bottom of the pot.)

Slowly add the beef broth and stir to loosen any flour that has stuck to the bottom of the pot. Once the flour has dissolved into the broth, add the tomato sauce, chili powder, paprika, and oregano. Stir until everything is evenly combined.

Add the pasta and stir to combine. Cover the pot, raise the heat to medium-high, and bring the mixture to a boil. Reduce the heat to low and simmer, stirring occasionally to prevent the pasta from sticking, for about 15 minutes, or until the pasta is tender and has absorbed most of the liquid. If the mixture becomes dry before the pasta has fully cooked, stir in an additional ¼ cup of water.

Remove the pot from the heat and stir in the cheese until it has melted. Serve hot.

 BUDGET BYTE Beef bouillon (cubes, granules, or beef base) reconstituted with water can be used in place of canned or boxed broth and will cost far less.

Greek Steak Tacos $$

Serves 4

Taco trucks are popping up all over the United States like little mobile weeds. Why? Because tacos are awesome and everyone knows it. Well, that, and because they're quick, easy, and fairly inexpensive. The most successful trucks break the taco mold by creating global fusion tacos with flavors from around the world. These Greek Steak Tacos are my take on that trend. Inexpensive flank steak is marinated in garlic and lemon, quickly seared, sliced thin, and then piled into tortillas. Like pico de gallo on a traditional taco, these tacos are topped with a fresh, Greek-inspired salad of tomato, red onions, and parsley. It's super easy, fresh, and flavorful . . . and you don't have to chase down a truck to get it.

FOR THE STEAK

- 1 (1¼-pound) flank or skirt steak
- 4 cloves garlic, minced
- 2 tablespoons olive oil
- 1 tablespoon lemon juice
- ½ teaspoon salt
- ½ teaspoon dried oregano
- Freshly cracked black pepper

FOR THE TOMATO SALAD

- 4 medium Roma tomatoes, diced small
- 1 small red onion, thinly sliced
- ½ bunch flat-leaf parsley, leaves only, roughly chopped
- 2 tablespoons olive oil
- 2 tablespoons lemon juice
- 1 teaspoon dried oregano
- ½ teaspoon salt

- 2 tablespoons vegetable oil
- 8 small flour tortillas

INSTRUCTIONS

Marinate the steak: Cut the flank steak into 2 or 3 pieces so that each is short enough to lie flat across the bottom of your largest skillet. Place the steak pieces in a large zip-top bag. Add the garlic, olive oil, lemon juice, salt, oregano, and 10 to 15 cranks of pepper. Seal the bag and massage the contents so that the steak is evenly coated in the marinade.

Allow the steak to marinate at room temperature for 30 minutes, or in the refrigerator for at least 30 minutes and up to 8 hours. If marinating in the refrigerator, allow the steak to come to room temperature before cooking, about 15 minutes. This will allow you to achieve a better sear on the meat.

Make the tomato salad: Place the tomato, onion, and parsley in a large bowl and toss to combine.

In a small bowl, whisk together the olive oil, lemon juice, oregano, and salt. Pour the dressing over the vegetables and stir to coat.

Cook the steak: In a large, heavy-bottomed skillet, heat 1 tablespoon of the vegetable oil over medium-high heat until shimmering, but not smoking. Add 1 piece of the flank steak and cook, without moving the steak, for 5 to 7 minutes. Once it is nicely browned on the bottom, flip it and cook, again without moving the steak, for 5 to 7 minutes more. The steak should be well browned on both sides, but still tender and pink in the center. Remove the steak and set aside on a cutting board. Add the remaining 1 tablespoon vegetable oil to the skillet and cook the remaining steak in the same manner.

Allow the steak to rest for 5 minutes before slicing. Slice the steak across the grain as thinly as possible. This will help make the meat more tender and easier to chew.

Pile a small amount of steak onto each tortilla and then top with an ample amount of the fresh tomato salad.

 Chef's Tip: Flank steak is one of the least expensive cuts of beef because it has more connective tissue and can be quite tough if not cooked correctly. Flank steak should only be cooked to medium-rare, or medium at most, to prevent it from becoming dry or leathery. Slicing the steak thinly and against the grain disrupts the connective tissue, making it even more tender.

Beef & Bean Taquitos $$

**Makes
12 taquitos**

These little taquitos are so much fun to eat. They make a great main dish or party appetizer and are a welcome change to chicken wings or takeout pizza for game-day get-
togethers. You can dip these taquitos in sour cream and salsa, or be the star of the show
and make your own Creamy Cilantro-Lime Dressing (page 71). Show up to a party with
homemade taquitos and creamy cilantro dipping sauce, and I guarantee you'll be invited
back to *every* party in the future.

INGREDIENTS

3 tablespoons vegetable oil

2 cloves garlic, minced

½ pound lean ground beef

1 (15-ounce) can black beans, drained
    and rinsed

½ tablespoon chili powder

½ teaspoon cornstarch

Pinch of cayenne pepper

¼ teaspoon salt

12 (6-inch) yellow corn tortillas

INSTRUCTIONS

Preheat the oven to 425°F. Line a rimmed baking sheet with foil.

In a large skillet, heat 1 tablespoon of the vegetable oil over medium heat. Add the garlic
and cook for 1 to 2 minutes, or until the garlic begins to soften. Add the ground beef and
continue to cook until the beef is thoroughly browned, 5 to 7 minutes.

Add the beans, chili powder, cornstarch, cayenne pepper, salt, and ½ cup of water to the
skillet and stir to combine. Bring the mixture to a simmer and cook for about 5 minutes,
or until the mixture is thick and bubbly. Mash the beans slightly while the mixture sim-
mers, as this will help hold the taquito filling together.

Stack the tortillas on a large plate and microwave for about 45 seconds, or until they are
hot, steamy, and very pliable. This will prevent the tortillas from splitting open as you
roll the taquitos.

Place about ¼ cup of the filling in each tortilla and roll the tortilla tightly into a cigar-shaped taquito. Place the rolled taquitos, seam side down, on the lined baking sheet.

Brush the remaining 2 tablespoons vegetable oil over the rolled taquitos, making sure to coat them well on all sides.

Bake the taquitos for 20 minutes, or until golden brown and crispy. Serve hot with salsa, sour cream, or Creamy Cilantro-Lime Dressing for dipping.

 BUDGET BYTE Because ground beef is not usually sold in ½-pound packages, I simply divide a 1-pound package in half and freeze the rest for use in another recipe. Just remember to label and date your freezer bags!

Spicy Beef 'n' Noodles $$

Serves 4
This Asian-inspired beef-noodle dish is a hybrid of two of the most popular recipes on my website, Dragon Noodles and Yakisoba. The rich, sweet, and spicy yakisoba sauce is combined with wide lo mein noodles and hearty ground beef for a dish that is nothing short of addictive. You'll have a hard time not going back for seconds with this one. Oh, and the best part? The beef cooks in about the same amount of time that it takes to boil the noodles, so you can have dinner ready in minutes!

INGREDIENTS

8 ounces wide lo mein noodles

1 tablespoon vegetable oil

1 clove garlic, minced

1-inch piece fresh ginger, peeled

½ pound lean ground beef

2 tablespoons soy sauce

2 tablespoons Worcestershire sauce

1 tablespoon ketchup

1 tablespoon sriracha

1 tablespoon brown sugar

2 green onions, sliced

Fresh cilantro (optional)

INSTRUCTIONS

Bring a large pot of water to a rolling boil. Add the lo mein noodles and cook for about 10 minutes, or until they are tender. Drain the cooked noodles in a colander.

While the noodles are cooking, in a large skillet, heat the vegetable oil over medium heat. Add the garlic and use a cheese grater or a Microplane to grate the ginger straight into the skillet. Sauté the garlic and ginger for about 2 minutes, or until they become soft and fragrant.

Add the ground beef to the skillet and cook until thoroughly browned, about 5 to 7 minutes.

In a small bowl, stir together the soy sauce, Worcestershire sauce, ketchup, sriracha, and brown sugar. Pour the sauce over the beef and cook for 3 to 5 minutes more, or until heated through. Add the cooked noodles and toss to coat in the sauce.

Sprinkle the green onions over the beef and noodles and top with fresh cilantro leaves, if desired.

BUDGET BYTE · Check Asian or ethnic markets for the best price on wide lo mein noodles. Although lo mein noodles have a uniquely delightful flavor and texture, fettuccine noodles can be substituted in a pinch.

Coconut Chicken Curry $$

Serves 6

I can't believe I used to hate curry. Maybe I tried it before I was ready. Maybe I hadn't acclimated myself to the heady spices of the East. Maybe it was just too different from the pizza and spaghetti that I was used to. That all changed when I had my first coconut curry. Coconut milk's gentle sweetness and creamy, rich texture help mellow out the exotic spices and make curry a little less intimidating.

This recipe takes advantage of a simple coconut curry sauce to add flavor and personality to an otherwise boring chicken breast, and rice helps bulk things up and keep costs low. Simple dishes like this have been keeping bellies full and mouths happy across the globe for generations.

INGREDIENTS

2 tablespoons vegetable oil

1 medium onion, diced

2 cloves garlic, minced

2-inch piece fresh ginger, peeled

1½ pounds boneless, skinless chicken breast, cut into 1½- to 2-inch chunks

½ teaspoon paprika

½ teaspoon ground turmeric

1 teaspoon hot or mild curry powder

2 (13.5-ounce) cans coconut milk

½ teaspoon salt

6 cups cooked rice

¼ bunch fresh cilantro, leaves only (optional)

INSTRUCTIONS

In a large pot, heat the vegetable oil over medium-low heat. Add the onion and garlic and, using a small-holed cheese grater or a Microplane, grate the ginger straight into the pot. Sauté for about 5 minutes, or until the onions are soft and translucent.

Add the chicken to the pot, raise the heat to medium, and continue to sauté until the chicken is cooked through, 7 to 10 minutes.

Add the paprika, turmeric, and curry powder and sauté for 1 minute more. Add the coconut milk and stir, scraping up any browned bits stuck to the bottom of the pot. Reduce the heat to low and cook for 10 minutes more, or until warmed through. Stir in the salt; taste the sauce and adjust the salt, if needed.

To serve, place 1 cup of the cooked rice in each of 6 bowls and then spoon the chicken and curry sauce over the top. Top with cilantro leaves, if desired.

 Chef's Tip: If you only have mild curry powder, you can make this dish spicy by adding ¼ teaspoon cayenne pepper.

 As always, seek out ethnic grocery stores for top-quality spices at the best prices.

Turkey Florentine Meatballs $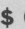

Serves 8

Meatballs are one of my favorite items to keep stocked in the freezer. I freeze the pre-cooked meatballs in single-serving portions, so that when I need a quick meal, I can just plop them into a pot of marinara sauce to reheat as the sauce warms. This version combines ground turkey, spinach, Parmesan, and plenty of herbs for an easy, flavorful fix.

INGREDIENTS

1 tablespoon vegetable oil

1 small onion, diced

2 cloves garlic, minced

1 (10-ounce) package frozen chopped spinach, thawed

1 (19-ounce) package ground turkey

1 large egg

¾ cup plain bread crumbs

½ cup grated Parmesan

½ teaspoon ground nutmeg

1 teaspoon dried oregano

½ teaspoon salt

INSTRUCTIONS

Preheat the oven to 375°F. Line a baking sheet with foil and coat it with nonstick cooking spray.

In a large skillet, heat the vegetable oil over medium-low heat. Add the onion and garlic and cook for about 5 minutes, or until the onion has softened.

Squeeze as much moisture as possible from the thawed spinach. Place the spinach in a large bowl and add the ground turkey, egg, bread crumbs, Parmesan, nutmeg, oregano, and salt. Add the sautéed onion and garlic and mix everything together until evenly combined. Your hands are the best tool for this job, but do not overmix or the meatballs will be tough.

Scoop tablespoons of the turkey mixture and roll them into balls slightly smaller than a Ping-Pong ball. The meatball mix should yield approximately 32 meatballs of this size.

Place the meatballs on the baking sheet and bake for 30 minutes, or until golden brown and crispy on the edges.

 Chef's Tip: Serve as an appetizer with toothpicks and marinara dipping sauce, or add the cooked meatballs to your favorite marinara and serve over pasta.

Chicken Tamale Pie

Serves 8

I love, love, *love* this dish. Flavorful, filling, and a breeze to pull together. Cooking the chicken right in a pot of homemade enchilada sauce gives the chicken extra flavor and a super-tender texture. Beans and corn bulk out the pie and add that classic Southwest flavor. A sweet-and-spicy jalapeño cornbread tops everything off and soaks up all of that wonderful enchilada sauce. This is one of those recipes that will make you jump for joy that you're eating leftovers.

INGREDIENTS

2 tablespoons vegetable oil

2 tablespoons all-purpose flour

2 tablespoons chili powder

¼ cup tomato paste

½ teaspoon ground cumin

½ teaspoon garlic powder

¼ teaspoon cayenne pepper

1 large boneless, skinless chicken
  breast (about ¾ pound), cut into
  1-inch cubes

1 (15-ounce) can black beans, drained
  and rinsed

1 cup frozen corn kernels

½ teaspoon salt

1 recipe Jalapeño Cornbread batter
  (page 45), unbaked

INSTRUCTIONS

In a medium saucepan, combine the vegetable oil, flour, and chili powder and whisk them together. Set the pan over medium heat and cook until the mixture begins to bubble. Continue to cook and whisk for 1 minute more.

Whisk in the tomato paste, cumin, garlic powder, cayenne pepper, and 1½ cups of water. Bring the mixture to a simmer; it will thicken slightly.

Add the cubed chicken to the sauce, making sure the pieces are mostly submerged under the sauce. Cover the pan and bring the mixture back to a simmer. Reduce the heat to low and continue to simmer for 30 minutes. Use two forks to shred or break up the chicken pieces in the sauce. Add the black beans, corn kernels, and salt to the pot with the chicken and sauce. Stir to combine.

Preheat the oven to 425°F.

Pour the chicken mixture into an 8-by-8-inch casserole dish or a 10-inch cast-iron skillet. Pour the Jalapeño Cornbread batter over the chicken mixture in the casserole dish, making sure to cover it evenly.

Bake for 25 minutes or until the top of the cornbread is golden brown on the edges and the sauce is bubbling up from below. Cut the casserole into 8 pieces and serve.

 Chef's Tip: This recipe is fairly spicy, but it can be made mild by simply leaving out the cayenne pepper from the enchilada sauce and the jalapeños from the cornbread.

Serves 4

Want to know a cheat to making food delicious? Roast it. Roasting makes almost anything better. The best part about roasting is that the oven does all the work. Just toss your ingredients together with a little oil and seasoning, pop them in the oven, and wait for the magic to happen. Roasting caramelizes sugars, deepens flavors, and creates tender textures. Meat and vegetables alike benefit from this technique, which is so simple, it feels like cheating.

This recipe uses a basic marinade with a classic combination of rosemary and garlic. The chicken and potatoes cook together in the same casserole dish, making prep even easier.

INGREDIENTS

¼ cup olive oil

¼ cup vegetable oil

4 cloves garlic, minced

1 tablespoon dried rosemary

2 teaspoons red wine vinegar

2 teaspoons salt

Freshly cracked black pepper

2 pounds bone-in, skin-on chicken pieces (thighs, drumsticks, or breasts)

2 pounds red potatoes, cubed

INSTRUCTIONS

Preheat the oven to 400°F. Coat a 9-by-13-inch casserole dish with nonstick cooking spray.

Combine the olive oil, vegetable oil, garlic, rosemary, vinegar, salt, and some pepper in a blender. Blend the mixture until smooth.

Place the chicken pieces in a zip-top bag and add half of the blended marinade. Seal the bag and massage the contents to distribute the marinade over the surface of the chicken. Refrigerate the chicken while you prepare the rest of the ingredients, or for up to 8 hours.

Place the cubed potatoes in the prepared casserole dish, pour the remaining marinade over the top, and toss until the potatoes are well coated with marinade.

Remove the marinated chicken pieces from the bag and nestle them down into the potatoes, skin side up. Pour any remaining marinade from the bag over the dish.

Roast for 45 to 50 minutes, or until the chicken skin is golden brown and crispy.

 Chef's Tip: For extra flavor, combine the chicken and marinade before work in the morning so that the flavors have all day to infuse into the chicken. Save the second half of the marinade in the refrigerator and add it to the potatoes just before roasting.

Teriyaki Chicken Sliders $$

Serves 4

This is my "quickie" version of a slow-cooker classic, because sometimes thinking ahead to use the slow cooker just doesn't happen. A short thirty-minute simmer in this home-made teriyaki sauce is enough to make the chicken tender, shreddable, and perfect for piling on a soft bun. The meat is then topped with chunks of pineapple to provide that salty-sweet contrast that we all love.

INGREDIENTS

¼ cup soy sauce

2 tablespoons rice vinegar

2 tablespoons brown sugar

2 cloves garlic, minced

2-inch piece fresh ginger, peeled

1 tablespoon vegetable oil

1 (20-ounce) can pineapple chunks
   in juice

1½ pounds boneless, skinless chicken
   breast, cut into 2-inch pieces

1 tablespoon cornstarch

4 soft rolls or hamburger buns

INSTRUCTIONS

In a medium saucepan, combine the soy sauce, vinegar, brown sugar, and garlic. Using a small-holed cheese grater or Microplane, grate the ginger straight into the pan. Strain the juice from the canned pineapple (about 1 cup) into the pan, reserving the pineapple pieces. Cook over medium heat, stirring, for about 5 minutes, or until the brown sugar has dissolved.

Place the chicken pieces in a single layer across the bottom of the pan, making sure they are submerged beneath the liquid.

Cover the pan, raise the heat to high, and bring the liquid to a boil. Reduce the heat to medium-low, uncover the pan, and simmer for 30 minutes, until reduced by about half. Stir the chicken pieces once or twice while simmering to keep them submerged in the liquid.

Use two forks to carefully shred the chicken in the pan. Combine the cornstarch with just enough water (about 2 tablespoons) to create a slurry and pour it into the pan. Stir to combine, raise the heat to medium, and bring the mixture back to a simmer; the sauce will thicken as it cooks.

Scoop one-quarter of the mixture onto each bun and top with a few of the reserved pineapple chunks.

Chorizo–Sweet Potato Enchiladas $

Serves 10

This recipe has a surprisingly bold flavor despite having only a few ingredients. How is that possible? Chorizo! Mexican chorizo is a full-flavored, spicy pork sausage that pairs perfectly with mild and creamy sweet potatoes. As if that wasn't enough to make your mouth water, go one step further and smother them in homemade enchilada sauce topped with melty cheese. Everyone will show up for dinner on time when it's Chorizo–Sweet Potato Enchilada night.

INGREDIENTS

2 tablespoons vegetable oil

1 medium sweet potato, peeled and cut into ½-inch cubes

1 medium poblano pepper, stemmed, seeded, and cut into ½-inch dice

2 cloves garlic, minced

¾ pound Mexican chorizo, casings removed (if links) (see Chef's Tip, at right)

10 (8-inch) flour tortillas

1 recipe Red Enchilada Sauce (page 77)

1½ cups shredded cheddar

3 to 4 green onions, sliced

INSTRUCTIONS

Preheat the oven to 375°F. Coat a 9-by-13-inch casserole dish with nonstick cooking spray.

In a large skillet, heat the vegetable oil over medium heat. Add the sweet potato, poblano pepper, and garlic and sauté for about 10 minutes, or until the sweet potato begins to soften. Add the chorizo and continue to cook, breaking up the sausage with a wooden spoon as it cooks, until it is fully browned, about 10 minutes.

Scoop about ¾ cup of the chorizo–sweet potato filling into each tortilla. Fold in the sides and roll the tortilla up around the filling like a burrito. Place the rolled enchiladas in the prepared casserole dish, seam side down.

Pour the enchilada sauce over the enchiladas and top them evenly with the shredded cheese. Bake for 20 minutes or until the cheese has melted and the sauce is hot and bubbly.

Sprinkle the green onions over the enchiladas before serving.

Chef's Tip: It's important to use Mexican chorizo instead of Spanish chorizo for this recipe. Mexican chorizo is a fresh meat product that is soft and can be sold either in links or as loose ground meat. Spanish chorizo is a cured meat product that is hard, dry, and often served sliced like pepperoni or salami.

Chef's Tip: Poblano peppers are a mild variety of pepper that boasts a unique flavor. You can recognize poblanos in the supermarket by their large size and dark green, waxy skin.

Five-Spice Chops $$

Serves 4 Chinese five-spice powder is my new secret weapon. It's an intoxicating blend of cinnamon, black pepper, ginger, fennel, and aniseed. It's savory and sweet all at the same time and will give incredible flavor and aroma to anything you cook. I paired it here with just a little garlic and brown sugar to further emphasize the savory-sweet combination, and cooked the chops quickly in a skillet to keep them juicy and tender.

INGREDIENTS

¼ cup brown sugar

1 tablespoon Chinese five-spice powder

½ teaspoon garlic powder

½ teaspoon salt

4 boneless thick-cut pork chops
   (about 1¼ pounds)

2 tablespoons vegetable oil

INSTRUCTIONS

In a small bowl, combine the brown sugar, five-spice powder, garlic powder, and salt and stir until blended.

Coat each pork chop generously with the five-spice rub on all sides. The residual moisture on the chops should moisten the rub and help it adhere to the meat.

In a large skillet, heat the vegetable oil over medium heat until shimmering. Add the chops to the skillet and cook until they are deep golden brown on each side, about 7 minutes per side. Cut one of the chops open to make sure they have cooked through and are no longer pink on the inside. If not cooked through, cover the skillet and continue to cook for 2 to 3 minutes more on each side.

BUDGET BYTE Chinese five-spice powder can be found in either the spice aisle or international foods section of most major grocery stores, but you'll find better prices at Asian or ethnic markets.

Herb-Roasted Pork Loin $$

Roasting wins again. You can turn a run-of-the-mill pork loin into a fancy-schmancy entrée with this simple technique that anyone can master, and you'll be blown away by the big flavor created with just a few herbs and some time in the oven. If you need something to impress a date, your in-laws, boss, or heck, even yourself (you're worth it), this recipe is it.

Serves 4

INGREDIENTS

2 cloves garlic

1 teaspoon dried basil

1 teaspoon dried thyme

1 teaspoon dried rosemary

½ teaspoon salt

Freshly cracked black pepper

2 tablespoons olive oil

1 (18- to 20-ounce) pork loin

INSTRUCTIONS

Preheat the oven to 425°F. Line a baking sheet with foil.

Combine the garlic, basil, thyme, rosemary, salt, and some pepper in a small food processor or blender. Process the mixture until the garlic is minced. (Alternatively, mince the garlic with a knife, roughly chop the rosemary, and stir them together with the basil, thyme, salt, and pepper.) Add the olive oil to the herb mixture and stir until combined.

Place the pork loin on the lined baking sheet and spread the herb mixture all over the surface of the pork loin, including the bottom side.

Bake for 40 minutes, or until a meat thermometer inserted in the thickest part of the pork loin registers 145°F. Remove the pork loin from the oven and transfer it to a cutting board to rest for 10 minutes before slicing.

BUDGET BYTE When shopping for your pork loin, pay special attention to the label. Pork loin is larger and less expensive than pork *tender*loin, which can cost two to three dollars more per pound.

 BUDGET BYTE A simple meat thermometer is an indispensable kitchen tool, and the most basic models can be purchased for just a few dollars. They take the guesswork out of cooking meat and will keep you (and your guests) happy and healthy.

Pork with Balsamic-Cranberry Sauce $$$

Serves 4

"Oooh, fancy pants!" That's what your friends will say when you bring this dish to the table. It looks and tastes like a million bucks, but is surprisingly simple and affordable. Pork tenderloin is tender and succulent, and is a blank slate for whatever indulgent sauce you want to drizzle over it. The quick cranberry pan sauce is the star of the show with its rich, sweet, and tangy flavor.

Pork tenderloin *is* one of the pricier cuts of meat, so keep this recipe tucked away for a special occasion. Pull out that bottle of wine you've been saving, whip up this pork tenderloin, and pretend that the world revolves around you for just one night. Not into pork? This sauce goes great over grilled chicken, too!

INGREDIENTS

1½ pounds pork tenderloin

2 cloves garlic, minced

2 tablespoons olive oil

2 tablespoons balsamic vinegar

⅛ teaspoon salt

Freshly cracked black pepper

1 (14-ounce) can whole-berry
cranberry sauce

¼ cup balsamic vinegar

1 tablespoon salted butter

½ teaspoon dried sage

INSTRUCTIONS

Place the pork in a large zip-top bag. Add the garlic, olive oil, balsamic vinegar, salt, and some pepper and seal the bag. Massage the contents to mix them and coat the pork in the marinade. Refrigerate the pork in the marinade for 30 minutes.

Preheat the oven to 425°F. Line a baking sheet with foil.

Heat a large skillet over medium-high heat. Add the pork and cook until it is deep golden brown on each side, about 7 minutes per side. Transfer the pork to the lined baking sheet and place it in the oven. Roast for 30 minutes, or until a meat thermometer inserted in the thickest part of the tenderloin registers 145°F.

In the same skillet used to brown the pork, add the cranberry sauce, balsamic vinegar, butter, and dried sage. Bring to a simmer over medium-low heat, whisking to combine. Simmer, using the whisk to help scrape up any browned bits from the bottom of the skillet, for about 10 minutes.

Remove the pork from the oven and transfer it to a cutting board to rest for about 10 minutes before slicing. Slice the pork and smother the pieces in the balsamic-cranberry sauce.

 Chef's Tip: Allowing the meat to rest before slicing helps keep it moist. When meat is fresh out of the oven the protein fibers are tightly contracted and most of the moisture is in the form of steam. This creates a high-pressure environment that causes moisture to escape quickly when the meat is sliced open. Giving the meat a few minutes to rest allows the meat fibers to relax, the steam pressure to reduce, and the juices to redistribute throughout the meat, where they are more likely to remain after the meat is sliced.

Asian Pork Lettuce Wraps $$

Those little Asian lettuce wraps that you get at the restaurant are *so* easy to make at home! It's as simple as cooking the rice, browning the meat, and adding a little seasoning. Having a "make your own" lettuce wrap night is a fun alternative to taco night and is a great idea for parties or small get-togethers. Just prepare the meat, set out the lettuce leaves and the toppings, and let the hungry eaters loose!

Makes 8 wraps

Most lettuce wrap recipes use Boston or butter lettuce because it's tender yet strong, but I've had great success using iceberg lettuce, which is not only less expensive, but also offers a nice crunch.

INGREDIENTS

1 tablespoon vegetable oil

1 pound ground pork

2 cloves garlic, minced

2-inch piece fresh ginger, peeled and grated

2 tablespoons soy sauce

2 tablespoons rice vinegar

2 tablespoons sugar

½ teaspoon toasted sesame oil

⅛ teaspoon red pepper flakes (optional)

1 (5-ounce) can sliced water chestnuts, drained and roughly chopped

1 head iceberg lettuce

2 cups cooked jasmine rice

2 medium carrots, grated

3 green onions, thinly sliced

INSTRUCTIONS

In a large skillet, heat the vegetable oil over medium heat. Add the ground pork and sauté until the pork is cooked through, 5 to 7 minutes. Drain off any excess fat from the pan.

Add the garlic and ginger to the skillet and continue to cook for 2 to 3 minutes more, or until the garlic has softened.

In a small bowl, combine the soy sauce, vinegar, sugar, sesame oil, and red pepper flakes, if using. Add the mixture to the skillet and stir to coat the pork in the sauce. Add the water chestnuts to the skillet.

Carefully remove the individual leaves from the head of lettuce. If any of the leaves are very large or wide, tear them in half to make two smaller pieces.

Spoon a couple of tablespoons of cooked rice into each lettuce leaf, followed by a couple of tablespoons of the pork mixture. Top with a sprinkle of grated carrot and sliced green onions. Fold the lettuce leaves over the ingredients and enjoy.

 Chef's Tip: Although jasmine rice offers a nice flavor, it is not a main player in this recipe and can be substituted with plain long-grain white rice.

Teriyaki Salmon with Sriracha Mayo $$$

Salmon is pretty pricey, so it isn't something that I get to enjoy often, but when I do, this *Serves 4* is my absolute favorite way to prepare it. The teriyaki marinade makes a perfectly flavorful exterior, while the inside of the salmon retains its mild and creamy flavor. The cooking method is brief, which ensures that the salmon stays moist and tender. A dollop of spicy sriracha mayonnaise on top creates a wonderful contrast to the sweet teriyaki sauce.

INGREDIENTS

¼ cup soy sauce

½ tablespoon toasted sesame oil

2 tablespoons brown sugar

2 tablespoons rice wine

1 teaspoon cornstarch

1 clove garlic, minced

1-inch piece fresh ginger, peeled

1 pound salmon fillet, skin on

2 tablespoons vegetable oil

¼ cup mayonnaise

2 tablespoons sriracha

INSTRUCTIONS

In a small bowl, stir together the soy sauce, sesame oil, brown sugar, rice wine, cornstarch, garlic, and 2 tablespoons of water. Using a small-holed cheese grater or a Microplane, grate the ginger straight into the bowl. Stir to combine.

Cut the salmon fillet into 4 equal-size pieces. Place them in a large zip-top bag and add the marinade. Squeeze out as much air as possible from the bag and seal it. Place the bag in the refrigerator and let the salmon marinate for 30 minutes.

In a large skillet, heat the vegetable oil over medium heat until it is shimmering. Add the fish and cook until it is nicely browned on all sides, 2 to 3 minutes per side.

In a small bowl, combine the mayonnaise and sriracha. Drizzle the mayonnaise mixture over the cooked fish just before serving.

Chef's Tip: Sriracha is a fiery Vietnamese hot sauce that has taken the culinary world by storm. It can be found in most major supermarkets and often goes by the nickname "rooster sauce" because of the rooster found on the label of the most popular brand.

Lemon-Garlic Shrimp Pasta $$

Serves 4

Shrimp are a wonderful treat, but they don't come cheap. So, to make this dish a little more budget friendly, we streeeetch it out with some inexpensive pasta and use simple ingredients, like lemon and garlic, to add flavor. This recipe is similar to a classic shrimp scampi, but for a fraction of the price that you'd pay at a restaurant. There's never been a better excuse to have date night at home than this mouthwatering Lemon-Garlic Shrimp Pasta.

INGREDIENTS

8 ounces linguine

2 tablespoons olive oil

2 tablespoons salted butter

2 cloves garlic, finely chopped

½ pound (41- to 50-count) peeled and deveined shrimp

1 medium lemon

Freshly cracked black pepper

Pinch of cayenne pepper (optional)

¼ bunch fresh flat-leaf parsley, roughly chopped

INSTRUCTIONS

Bring a large pot of salted water to a rolling boil. Add the pasta and cook for 7 to 10 minutes, or just until the pasta is tender. Drain and set aside.

In a large skillet, heat the olive oil and butter over medium heat until the butter is melted. Add the garlic and sauté for 2 to 3 minutes, or until the garlic is tender.

Rinse the shrimp under cool water and drain them. Add the shrimp to the skillet and sauté for about 5 minutes, or until the shrimp are opaque.

Using a Microplane or a small-holed cheese grater, scrape off the thin yellow layer of zest from the lemon (do not grate down to the white pith). Juice the lemon into a small bowl.

Add the lemon zest and lemon juice to the shrimp in the skillet and season with black pepper and a pinch of cayenne pepper, if desired.

Add the cooked pasta and toss to coat the pasta in the sauce. Sprinkle the parsley over the pasta and serve hot.

 Chef's Tip: You can use either fresh or frozen shrimp for this recipe. If using frozen shrimp, simply thaw them by placing them in the refrigerator a day ahead of time or place the frozen shrimp in a colander and run cool water over them until thawed. Do not let the shrimp sit in stagnant water to thaw as this can be a food safety hazard.

Thai Steamed Fish $$$

Serves 2

This fish is quick, fresh, and exotic. It's a breeze to pull together, bakes in twenty short minutes, and tastes like a meal at a fancy Thai restaurant. Fish sauce is the star ingredient, so don't be tempted to skip it. You can find fish sauce in the Asian section of most major grocery stores or in any Asian market. Fish sauce is extremely potent, so you won't want to taste or smell it straight. Only a small amount is needed to add a ton of savory flavor to any dish.

Parchment squares folded into packets hold in moisture and steam the fish while it bakes. You can eat the steamed fish straight out of the parchment packet for a low-carb meal, or serve it over a bowl of hot jasmine rice, making sure to spoon the cooking juices over the top.

INGREDIENTS

1 medium red bell pepper, julienned

1 medium zucchini, julienned

2 (3-ounce) white fish fillets
    (cod, mahi-mahi, sea bass)

1 clove garlic, minced

1 teaspoon fish sauce

1 tablespoon rice vinegar

1 tablespoon honey

⅛ teaspoon red pepper flakes

Juice of ½ small lime

1 green onion, sliced

Fresh cilantro sprigs

INSTRUCTIONS

Preheat the oven to 400°F. Tear off 2 large pieces of parchment paper, approximately 18 by 18 inches each. Place the parchment squares side by side on a large baking sheet.

Place a handful of the bell pepper and a handful of the zucchini in the center of each parchment paper square. Place a fish fillet on top of each pile of vegetables.

In a small bowl, combine the garlic, fish sauce, vinegar, honey, red pepper flakes, and lime juice and stir to combine. Spoon half of the sauce over each piece of fish. Sprinkle the green onion slices over each piece of fish.

Fold the parchment paper into a packet: Bring the top and bottom edges of the parchment square up to meet in the center. Fold them down tightly multiple times until the fold comes to about 1 inch above the surface of the fish. Take the 2 open sides of the parchment packet and fold them under multiple times, until the folds come within about 1 inch of the sides of the fish. Repeat with the second piece of parchment paper.

Transfer the baking sheet to the oven and bake for 20 minutes. To serve, carefully open the packets and top with a few sprigs of fresh cilantro. Serve the fish in the parchment paper packet or transfer the entire contents (including juices) over a bowl of cooked jasmine rice.

Nine

RICE, BEANS & LENTILS

Rice, beans, and lentils are staple ingredients in my kitchen. They are inexpensive, healthy, and have an almost endless shelf life when stored in airtight containers, away from heat and moisture. The trick is learning how to spruce them up into something that will keep you coming back for more. On their own, rice, beans, and lentils can be boring, but the sky is the limit when it comes to seasoning. So let's get creative and discover just how amazing and versatile they can be!

Taco Rice   *180*

Savory Coconut Rice   *181*

Cilantro-Lime Rice   *182*

Pineapple Fried Rice   *183*

Quick Chipotle Black Beans   *184*

Spiced Chickpeas   *185*

Autumn Lentil Pilaf   *186*

White Beans with Spinach & Bacon   *188*

Southwest Veggie & Rice Casserole   *190*

Tuscan White Beans   *192*

Calico Beans   *193*

Emerald Rice Salad   *195*

Taco Rice

Serves 6

Why have plain white rice when you can have taco rice instead? Taco rice slices, it dices, it juliennes . . . okay, maybe not, but it *does* have many different uses. Eat it as a side dish, stuff it into a burrito, use it as a base for a bean-and-rice bowl, or use it as a base for a casserole, like in my Southwest Veggie & Rice Casserole (page 190). Taco rice doesn't take much more time than cooking regular white rice, but has so much more to brag about.

INGREDIENTS

½ tablespoon chili powder

½ teaspoon ground cumin

½ teaspoon garlic powder

¼ teaspoon dried oregano

1 teaspoon salt

2 tablespoons tomato paste

2 cups long-grain white rice

INSTRUCTIONS

In a medium saucepan, whisk together the chili powder, cumin, garlic powder, oregano, salt, tomato paste, and 3 cups of water.

Add the rice and stir briefly to combine. Cover the pan, raise the heat to high, and bring to a full boil. Reduce the heat to low and simmer for 20 minutes.

Remove the pan from the heat and let the rice stand, undisturbed, for 20 minutes more.

Remove the lid, fluff the rice with a fork, and serve.

 Chef's Tip: For extra flavor, use chicken broth in place of water. Chicken broth already contains salt, so you will not need the teaspoon of salt listed in the ingredients.

Savory Coconut Rice $ ❄

This is my "go-to" side dish for most Asian meals. It's so good that just the smell of it *Serves 6* makes my mouth water. The combination of fragrant jasmine rice, rich coconut milk, and savory garlic creates a heady yet mild rice that will add extra pizzazz to your meal. Serve it as a side or use it as bed for my Teriyaki Salmon with Sriracha Mayo (page 173) or even my Five-Spice Chops (page 166).

Using jasmine rice really is key, so don't be tempted to substitute plain white rice. For the best price on jasmine rice, shop Asian markets, check bulk bins, or the bottom shelf in the rice or international foods aisle, where large five-pound bags of jasmine rice often hide.

INGREDIENTS

1½ cups jasmine rice

1 (15-ounce) can coconut milk

1 clove garlic, minced

¾ teaspoon salt

INSTRUCTIONS

In a medium saucepan, combine the rice, coconut milk, garlic, salt, and 1 cup of water and stir to combine. Cover the pan, raise the heat to high, and bring the mixture to a boil. Reduce the heat to low and simmer for 20 minutes.

Remove the pan from the heat and let the rice stand, undisturbed, for 20 minutes more.

Remove the lid, fluff the rice with a fork, and enjoy!

 Chef's Tip: This recipe can also be made in a rice cooker. Just place all the ingredients in the rice cooker and press go!

Cilantro-Lime Rice

Serves 6

This is another "must-have" rice recipe and one that works with just about any Southwest- or Tex-Mex-themed meal. It's simple to prepare and boasts big flavor. I like to eat this as a side dish, as the base for rice-and-bean bowls, or stuffed into burritos with black beans and seasoned beef, chicken, or pork. Fresh lime is critical to achieving the bright flavor, so don't be tempted to use bottled juice.

INGREDIENTS

2 cups long-grain white rice

3 cups chicken broth

1 medium lime

½ bunch fresh cilantro, leaves only, roughly chopped

Salt (optional)

INSTRUCTIONS

In a medium saucepan, combine the rice and chicken broth. Cover the pan, raise the heat to high, and bring the mixture to a boil. Reduce the heat to low and simmer for 20 minutes.

Remove the pan from the heat and let the rice stand, undisturbed, for 20 minutes more.

Using a Microplane or a small-holed cheese grater, scrape off the thin green layer of zest from the lime (do not grate down to the white pith). Cut the lime in half and juice one half into a small bowl. Reserve the remaining half.

Remove the lid and fluff the rice with a fork. Stir in the cilantro, lime zest, and lime juice. Taste the rice and add more lime juice or salt, if desired.

Pineapple Fried Rice

The key to good fried rice is using day-old or cold rice. This keeps the rice grains separate and fluffy, rather that sticky and mushy. For that reason, this recipe is *perfect* for using up extra rice. So, never throw your leftover cooked rice away again—reuse and repurpose!

Serves 4

Although fried rice is often eaten as a side dish, you can make a meal out of it by adding shrimp, chicken, tofu, or cashews.

INGREDIENTS

2 tablespoons vegetable oil

1 clove garlic, minced

1 large egg

¼ cup frozen peas

1 (8-ounce) can crushed pineapple, drained

3 tablespoons soy sauce

1 teaspoon sugar

⅛ teaspoon red pepper flakes

3 cups cooked rice

½ teaspoon toasted sesame oil

2 green onions, sliced

¼ bunch fresh cilantro, leaves only (optional)

INSTRUCTIONS

In a large skillet, heat the vegetable oil over medium heat. Add the garlic and cook for 1 to 2 minutes, or just until the garlic begins to soften. Lightly whisk the egg in a bowl, then pour it into the skillet. Gently scramble the egg as it cooks. Add the peas and pineapple to the skillet.

In a small bowl, combine the soy sauce, sugar, and red pepper flakes. Pour the mixture over the ingredients in the skillet and stir to combine.

Add the cooked rice to the skillet, stir to combine, and cook for 5 to 7 minutes, or until heated through. Sprinkle the toasted sesame oil over the rice and gently stir to combine.

Sprinkle the sliced green onions and cilantro leaves, if using, over the rice and serve immediately.

Quick Chipotle Black Beans $

Serves
3 to 4

Chipotle peppers in adobo sauce instantly transform any dish into a deep, smoky, spicy delight. In this recipe, they turn a humble can of black beans into a super side dish worthy of any meal. Beware, though: This one is for heat seekers. Chipotle peppers are extremely spicy and even the small amount added in this recipe brings a considerable amount of heat!

INGREDIENTS

1 tablespoon vegetable oil

1 clove garlic, minced

1 (15-ounce) can black beans

½ teaspoon ground cumin

1 teaspoon brown sugar

1 (7-ounce) can chipotle peppers in
   adobo sauce (see Budget Byte, below)

INSTRUCTIONS

In a small saucepan, heat the vegetable oil over medium heat. Add the garlic and sauté for 1 to 2 minutes, or until the garlic begins to soften.

Add the black beans and their liquid, the cumin, and the brown sugar and stir to combine.

Take 1 chipotle pepper from the can, mince it, and add it to the beans. Scoop about 1 teaspoon of adobo sauce from the can and add it to the beans. Stir to combine and cook for 5 minutes, or until heated through.

 BUDGET BYTE Even though chipotle peppers in adobo sauce come in a very small can, I rarely use more than one pepper per recipe. The rest gets frozen in a small freezer bag for later use. You can also freeze them individually in an ice cube tray and then transfer them to a freezer bag for storage.

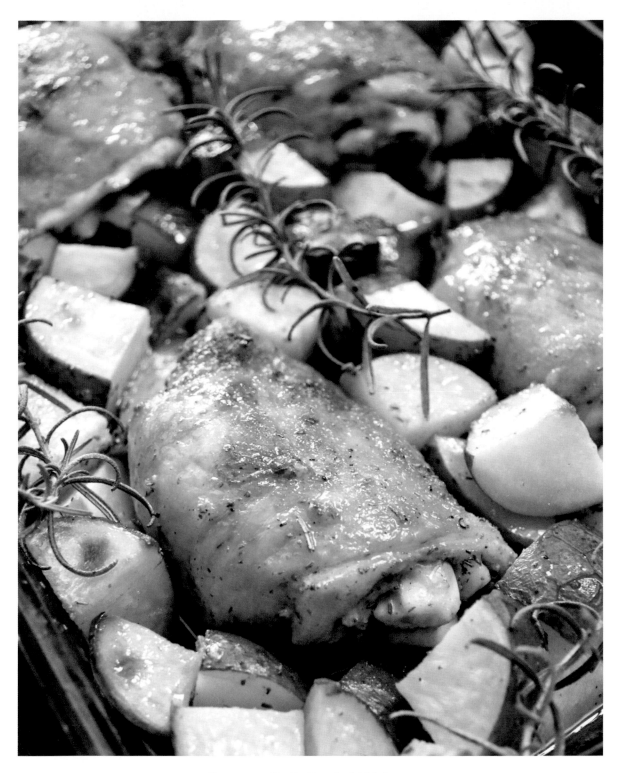

Rosemary-Garlic Roasted Chicken
& Potatoes, page 160

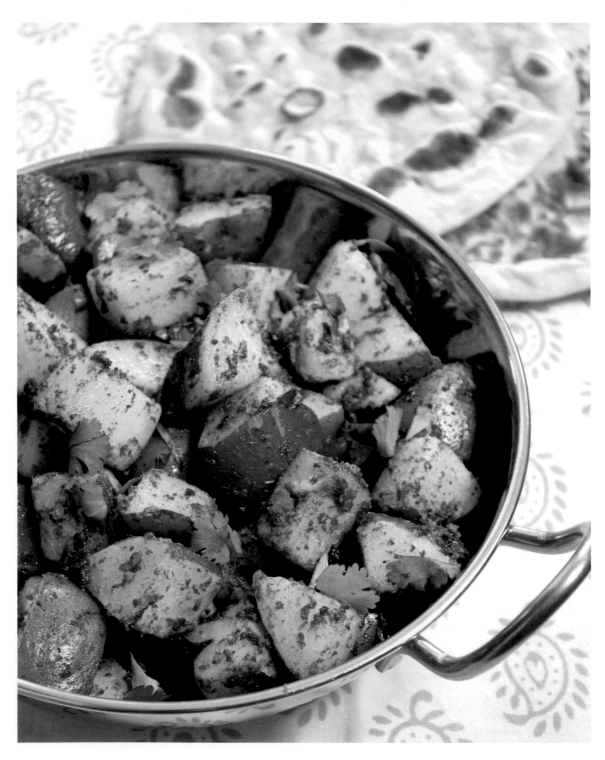

Indian Skillet Potatoes, page 203
with Naan, page 56

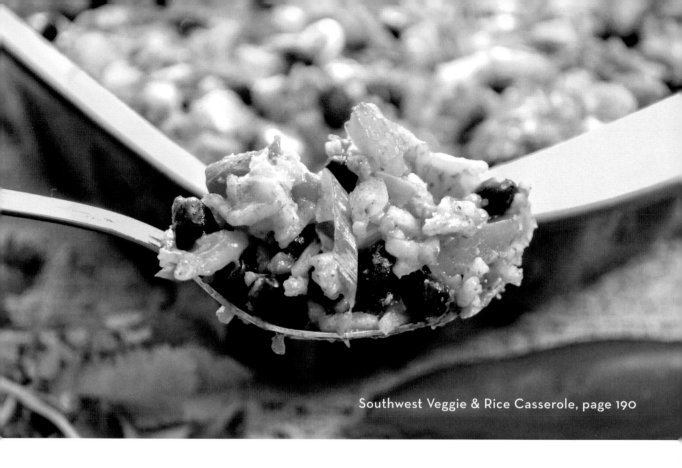

Southwest Veggie & Rice Casserole, page 190

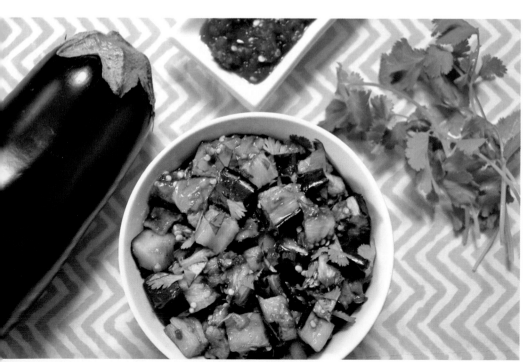

Spicy Roasted
Eggplant
page 201

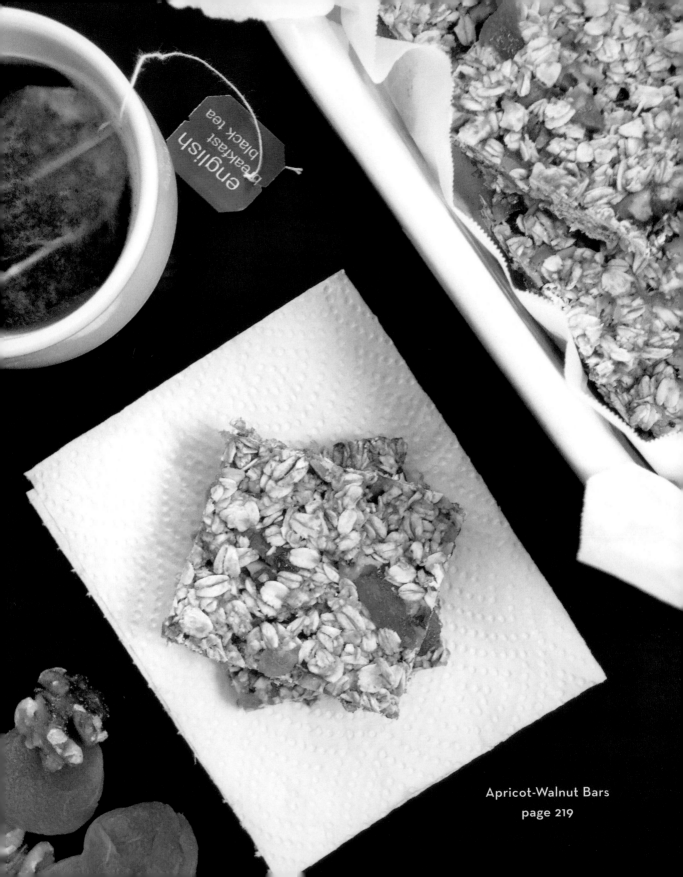

english breakfast black tea

Apricot-Walnut Bars
page 219

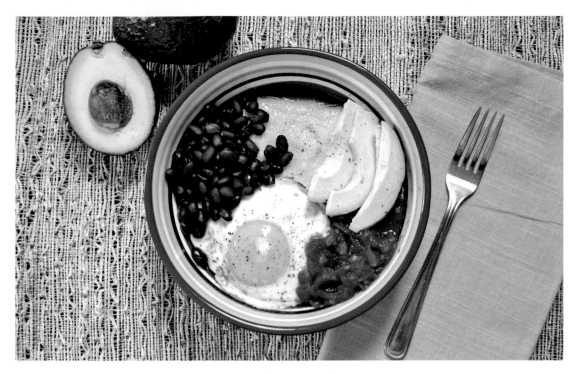

Huevos Rancheros Bowls, page 29

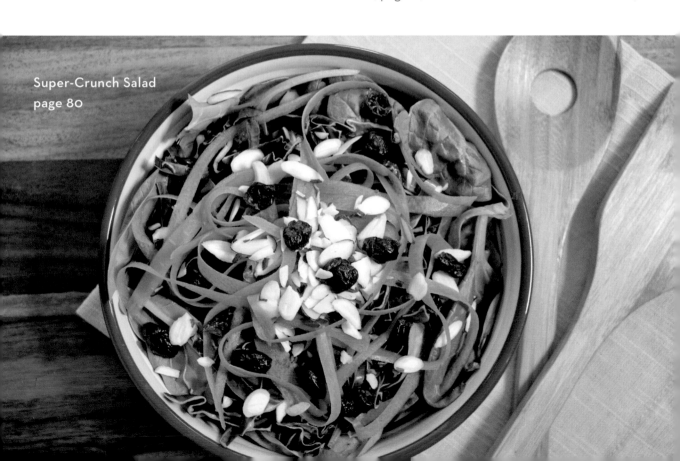

Super-Crunch Salad
page 80

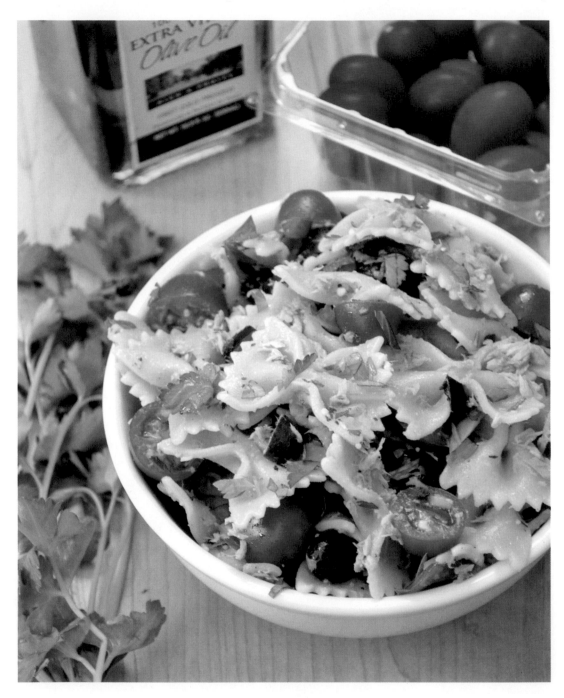

Pasta with Tuna & Olives

page 109

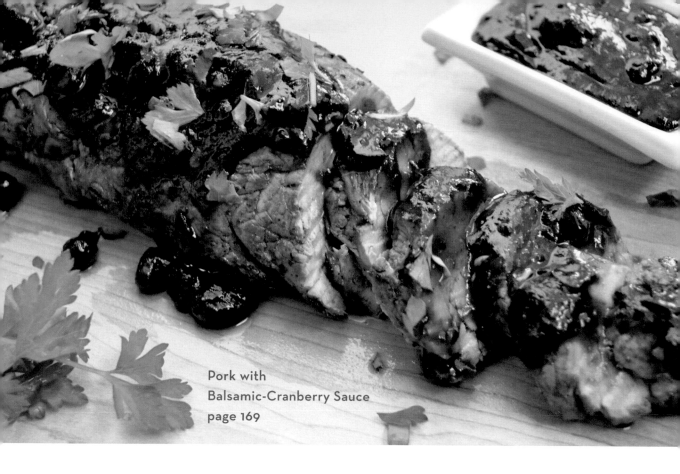

Pork with
Balsamic-Cranberry Sauce
page 169

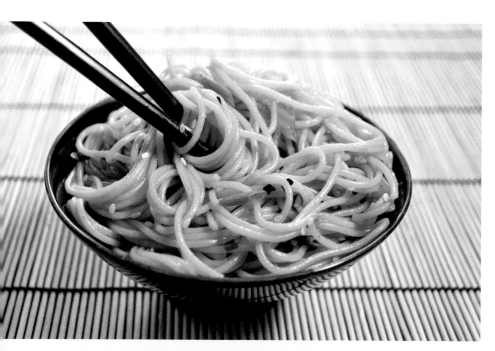

Sesame Noodles
page 114

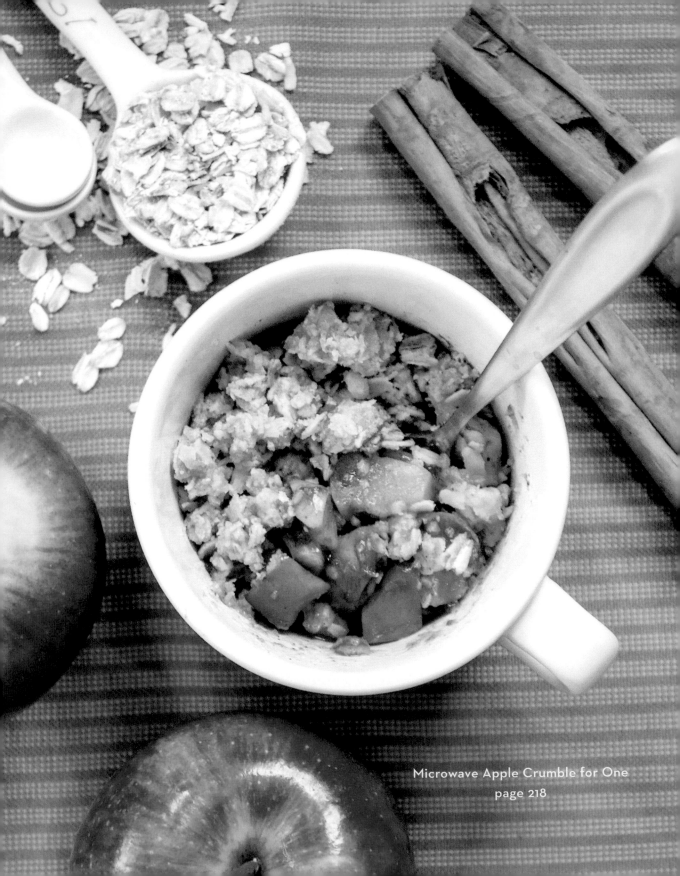

Microwave Apple Crumble for One
page 218

Spiced Chickpeas $

This is a super-fast way to take a plain can of chickpeas and turn them into something delicious and filling. They're smoky, spicy, a little sweet, and totally addictive. Serve these beans next to a hamburger, or with a rice pilaf and some hearty greens for a vegetarian meal. Play around with the spices to come up with your own unique mix!

Serves 6

INGREDIENTS

2 tablespoons olive oil

1 medium onion, diced

2 cloves garlic, minced

2 (15-ounce) cans chickpeas, drained
    and rinsed

1 teaspoon smoked paprika

1 teaspoon chili powder

½ teaspoon ground cumin

⅛ teaspoon cayenne pepper

1 teaspoon brown sugar

½ teaspoon salt

Freshly cracked black pepper

INSTRUCTIONS

In a large skillet, heat the olive oil over medium heat. Add the onion and garlic and cook for 5 to 7 minutes, or until the onions become golden brown on the edges. Add the chickpeas to the skillet.

In a small bowl, combine the smoked paprika, chili powder, cumin, cayenne pepper, brown sugar, salt, and a few cranks of a pepper mill. Sprinkle the spices over the chickpeas in the skillet and stir to combine. Cook for 5 minutes, or until heated through, and then serve.

Autumn Lentil Pilaf

Serves 4

Rice and lentils are a classic combination. Not only do they provide a complete protein, but they're easy to cook and can be seasoned any number of ways. This version is slightly sweet, slightly savory, and has the warm aromatic spices of autumn. To turn this from a savory side dish into a vegan entrée, simply add some walnuts for extra protein, texture, and flavor.

INGREDIENTS

1 tablespoon olive oil

½ medium onion, diced

½ cup white rice

½ teaspoon ground allspice

½ cup brown lentils

⅓ cup dried cranberries

½ teaspoon salt

¼ bunch fresh flat-leaf parsley, leaves only, roughly chopped

INSTRUCTIONS

In a medium saucepan, heat the olive oil over medium heat. Add the onion and cook for about 5 minutes, or until the onion is soft and translucent.

Add the rice and allspice to the pot and stir to combine. Cook, stirring, for 2 minutes to slightly toast the rice and allspice.

Add the lentils, cranberries, salt, and 1¾ cups of water to the pot and stir to combine. Cover the pot and raise the heat to high. Bring the mixture to a boil, then reduce the heat to low and simmer for 20 minutes.

Remove the pan from the heat and let stand, undisturbed, for 20 minutes more.

Remove the lid from the pan, fluff the rice and lentils with a fork, and fold in the parsley until evenly mixed. Serve hot.

Chef's Tip: Make sure to use brown lentils, which cook faster than green or French lentils. If the package does not specify, check the cooking instructions. Brown lentils take approximately 20 minutes to cook, while French lentils take closer to 45 minutes. Red and yellow lentils fall apart when cooked and are not well suited to this recipe.

White Beans with Spinach & Bacon $

Serves 4

This is one of those recipes that makes me want to throw my head back and scream, "I LOVE BEANS!" You might think that sounds extreme, but you haven't tried *these* beans. It's the perfect meal—creamy white beans, salty bacon, and fresh spinach make a well-rounded, colorful dish that can only be improved by the addition of crusty bread for dipping. It's super easy, whips up in a few minutes, and is light on the wallet. Beans: They're what's for dinner.

INGREDIENTS

3 ounces bacon (3 to 4 slices)

1 medium onion, diced

1 (15-ounce) can Great Northern beans, drained and rinsed

1 cup chicken broth

Freshly cracked black pepper

2 cups fresh baby spinach

INSTRUCTIONS

In a large skillet, cook the bacon over medium heat until crispy. Transfer the bacon to a paper towel–lined plate.

Pour out most of the bacon fat from the skillet, leaving 1 to 2 tablespoons behind. Return the skillet to the stovetop over medium heat and add the onion. Cook the onion for about 5 minutes, or until soft and translucent.

Add the beans and chicken broth and bring the mixture to a simmer. Simmer for about 10 minutes, or until the liquid has reduced by half and thickened. Season with pepper to taste.

Stir the spinach into the beans until it has wilted. Crumble the cooked bacon over the top and serve.

When fresh spinach is too pricey, substitute ½ pound frozen spinach. Try to use whole frozen spinach rather than chopped, to achieve a similar appearance.

 I often use small amounts of bacon to add a lot of flavor to dishes. Rather than cooking individual strips, I cut the package across the strips into four 3-ounce sections, which can then be frozen and thawed when needed.

 Chef's Tip: Never pour hot grease down the drain, as it can cause serious clogs. When pouring off grease from bacon or any other meat, pour it into a heat-proof dish or container and then wait until it cools and solidifies before scooping it into the garbage or saving it for later use (bacon grease is great for adding flavor!).

Southwest Veggie & Rice Casserole $$

Serves 8   I could eat a simple bowl of rice, black beans, salsa, and cheddar cheese any day, but this recipe takes that concept to the next level. Taco Rice (page 180) gives this casserole an ultra-flavorful base to build upon and a mélange of vegetables provides more texture and flavor than you can shake a maraca at. A little cheddar cheese thrown on top is like icing on the cake to this yummy Southwest casserole. So come on, get your veggie on!

INGREDIENTS

2 tablespoons vegetable oil

1 medium onion, diced

2 cloves garlic, minced

1 medium jalapeño, seeded and diced

1 medium bell pepper, seeded and diced

1 medium zucchini, quartered
    lengthwise and sliced

½ tablespoon chili powder

¾ teaspoon salt

1 cup frozen corn kernels

1 (15-ounce) can diced tomatoes with
    chiles (see Chef's Tip, below)

1 (15-ounce) can black beans,
    drained and rinsed

3 cups Taco Rice (page 180)

2 cups shredded sharp cheddar

2 green onions, thinly sliced

INSTRUCTIONS

Preheat the oven to 375°F. Coat an 8-by-8-inch casserole dish with nonstick cooking spray.

In a large skillet, heat the vegetable oil over medium-low heat. Add the onion and garlic and cook for about 5 minutes, or until the onions have softened. Add the jalapeño and bell peppers, zucchini, chili powder, and salt to the skillet and stir to combine. Raise the heat to medium and continue to sauté until the vegetables are soft and no liquid remains on the bottom of the skillet, about 10 minutes.

In a large bowl, combine the corn kernels, diced tomatoes and chiles, and black beans. Add the sautéed vegetables, Taco Rice, and shredded cheddar cheese to the bowl and stir until evenly mixed.

Pour the rice and vegetable mixture into the prepared casserole dish and bake for 20 minutes.

Sprinkle the green onions over the casserole and serve.

 Chef's Tip: If you are unable to find canned tomatoes with chiles, you can substitute one 15-ounce can regular diced tomatoes plus one 4-ounce can mild green chiles.

Serves 6

Savory herbs and tangy red wine vinegar transform a simple can of white beans into an ultra-flavorful, super-fast side dish. The flavor profile evokes dining at a Mediterranean tapas restaurant, except you won't be receiving a large check for a small portion (and thank goodness, because I want to eat them *all*). Serve these beans alongside roasted meats, or stuff them into a pita with tomato and fresh spinach for a light vegetarian meal.

INGREDIENTS

¼ cup olive oil

2 cloves garlic, minced

2 (15-ounce) cans white beans (cannellini or Great Northern), drained and rinsed

½ teaspoon dried thyme

½ teaspoon dried rosemary

½ teaspoon salt

Freshly cracked black pepper

1 tablespoon red wine vinegar

INSTRUCTIONS

In a large skillet, heat the olive oil over medium-low heat. Add the garlic and sauté for 1 to 2 minutes, or until the garlic just begins to soften.

Add the beans, thyme, rosemary, salt, a generous dose of pepper, and ½ cup of water and stir to combine. Raise the heat to medium, bring the mixture to a simmer, and cook for 10 minutes.

Stir in the red wine vinegar and serve.

Calico Beans

 $ ❄

Calico beans are a fun alternative to the traditional baked beans served with summertime *Serves 4* grilled meals. They're quick, colorful, and drenched in a sweet, tangy sauce. Although most calico bean recipes include ground beef, I find that a little bit of bacon and a splash of Worcestershire sauce add all the meaty flavor I need. Plus, the hearty mix of beans is plenty filling on its own!

INGREDIENTS

3 ounces bacon (3 to 4 slices), cut into small pieces

1 small onion, diced

¼ cup brown sugar

¼ cup tomato paste

3 tablespoons apple cider vinegar

1 tablespoon Dijon mustard

1 tablespoon Worcestershire sauce

½ teaspoon smoked paprika

½ teaspoon salt

Freshly cracked black pepper

1 (15-ounce) can kidney beans, drained and rinsed

1 (15-ounce) can white beans, drained and rinsed

1 (15-ounce) can lima beans, drained and rinsed

INSTRUCTIONS

In a large skillet, cook the bacon over medium heat for about 10 minutes, or until it is crispy and has rendered most of its fat. Pour off most of the fat in the pan, leaving about 2 tablespoons in the skillet.

Add the onion and sauté it in the bacon fat for about 5 minutes, or until the onion has softened.

Add the brown sugar, tomato paste, vinegar, mustard, Worcestershire sauce, paprika, salt, pepper, and ¼ cup of water to the skillet. Whisk to combine and dissolve any browned bits that may be stuck to the bottom of the skillet.

Add the beans to the skillet. Stir to combine with the sauce and cook for 5 to 7 minutes, or until heated through.

BUDGET BYTE Save your leftover tomato paste by spooning it into a small zip-top bag and popping it in the freezer. Don't forget to label and date the packages!

Chef's Tip: Never pour hot grease down your drain, as it can cause serious clogs. When pouring off grease from bacon or any other meat, pour it into a heatproof dish or container and then wait until it cools and solidifies before scooping it into the garbage or saving it for later use (bacon grease is great for adding flavor!).

Emerald Rice Salad $

Serves 4

This pretty green rice salad is delicious and simple to prepare. The beautiful emerald color comes from avocado, which also adds a creamy texture and flavor. Crushed pineapple adds just the right amount of sweetness, while grated ginger gives it a little zing. This rice can be eaten warm or cold and makes the perfect side dish to light summer meals or any Caribbean-inspired dishes.

INGREDIENTS

- 1 ripe medium avocado, diced
- 1 (15-ounce) can crushed pineapple, drained (reserve the juice for another use)
- 1-inch piece fresh ginger, peeled
- ¼ teaspoon salt
- 3 cups cooked long-grain white or jasmine rice, cooled slightly

INSTRUCTIONS

In a large bowl, combine the avocado and crushed pineapple. Using a small-holed cheese grater or a Microplane, grate the ginger straight into the bowl. Sprinkle the salt over the ingredients in the bowl.

Add the rice to the bowl and gently fold it into the avocado mixture, until everything is evenly mixed and the rice has taken on a light green hue. Serve warm or refrigerate until ready to eat.

Chef's Tip: A ripe avocado is essential for this recipe. An underripe avocado will not mix in properly with the rice. Look for an avocado that yields slightly when squeezed, but is not mushy.

BUDGET BYTE The leftover pineapple juice is excellent for use in smoothies or cocktails. If you can't use it immediately, it can be frozen for later use.

Ten

VEGETABLES

Vegetables make me excited. There are so many colors, textures, and flavors to play with that the possibilities are endless! If you have a picky eater who claims to dislike vegetables, there is a good chance that they just haven't had them prepared the right way. Vegetables can easily be overcooked or poorly seasoned, leaving a bland, mushy mess. Use the recipes in this chapter to learn how to add flavor and create texture when cooking vegetables. To keep costs in check, always choose vegetables that are in season or on sale. Frozen vegetables, which rarely have any added ingredients, can also be a very economical choice—just be sure to avoid frozen vegetables that come pre-seasoned or in a premade sauce.

Cumin-Lime Sweet Potato Sticks *198*

Roasted Broccoli with Crispy Garlic *199*

Spicy Roasted Eggplant *201*

Indian Skillet Potatoes *203*

Lemon-Butter Green Beans *204*

Italian Spaghetti Squash *205*

Firecracker Cauliflower *207*

Chipotle–Sweet Potato Quesadillas *208*

Ginger Snow Peas *210*

Triple-Herb Mashed Potatoes *211*

Roasted Carrots & Zucchini *213*

Cumin-Lime Sweet Potato Sticks $

Serves 4

Sweet potatoes are one of my favorite vegetables because they're filling, versatile, packed with flavor and nutrients, and super inexpensive. These uniquely seasoned fries were one of the first things I ever learned to make with sweet potatoes and I've been hooked ever since. The subtle sweetness of the potatoes is balanced with earthy cumin and a tart splash of lime juice. Although they're not crispy like a deep-fried French fry, the addictive flavor more than makes up for it!

INGREDIENTS

2 pounds sweet potatoes, peeled and cut into ½-inch-thick sticks

1 tablespoon olive oil

½ tablespoon ground cumin

1 teaspoon salt

¼ bunch fresh cilantro, leaves only, roughly chopped

1 medium lime

INSTRUCTIONS

Preheat the oven to 425°F. Line a rimmed baking sheet with parchment paper.

Place the sweet potato sticks in a large bowl. Add the olive oil, cumin, salt, and cilantro to the bowl. Toss until everything is well coated in oil and herbs.

Spread the sweet potatoes in a single layer on the lined baking sheet, using a second baking sheet if necessary to make sure the sweet potato sticks are not piled on top of one another.

Bake for 45 minutes, or until the potatoes are tender and slightly golden brown on the edges. Stir once halfway through.

Squeeze the juice from the lime over the sweet potato sticks and serve hot.

Roasted Broccoli with Crispy Garlic $

Roasting vegetables is one of the quickest ways to take vegetables from boring to ahhh-mazing. The slow-roasting process caramelizes their natural sugars and makes them slightly sweet, mild, and smoky. Broccoli in particular is one of my favorite vegetables to roast. The tender florets grab hold of any seasoning you add to them, ensuring that every bite is full of maximum flavor.

Serves 4

INGREDIENTS

1 bunch (2 crowns) broccoli

2 tablespoons olive oil

4 cloves garlic, minced

½ teaspoon salt

Freshly cracked black pepper

1 medium lemon (optional)

INSTRUCTIONS

Preheat the oven to 400°F. Line a rimmed baking sheet with foil or parchment paper.

Cut the broccoli into small florets, leaving 1 to 2 inches of stem attached to each floret. Place the cut broccoli in a large bowl.

Add the olive oil, garlic, and salt to the bowl with the broccoli and toss until the broccoli is well coated in oil. Try to work the minced garlic into the crevices of the florets.

Place the coated broccoli in a single layer on the lined baking sheet. Season lightly with pepper.

Roast for 30 minutes, stirring once halfway through.

If desired, squeeze the juice from the lemon over the broccoli before serving.

BUDGET BYTE Broccoli stems become tender and delicious when roasted, so try not to cut the florets off close to the top. Leave a couple of inches of stem attached and get more broccoli out of your bunch!

Chef's Tip: Although frozen broccoli is great for many recipes, it is too moist and soft for this recipe. You'll only achieve the deep roasted flavor and texture with fresh broccoli.

Spicy Roasted Eggplant $$

This Asian-inspired eggplant dish is absolutely addictive. Eggplant may be spongy and bitter when raw, but it roasts down to a creamy delicacy. The skin and seeds offer just enough texture to keep it from being too mushy, while the rich and spicy sauce teases your taste buds. Oyster sauce, which can be found in the Asian section of most grocery stores, is the perfect savory base for this spicy sauce.

Serves 4

INGREDIENTS

2 medium eggplants (about 1½ pounds), cut into 1-inch cubes

3 tablespoons olive oil

½ teaspoon salt

3 tablespoons oyster sauce

3 tablespoons chili garlic sauce

¾ teaspoon sugar

¼ bunch cilantro, leaves only (optional)

Cooked rice, for serving (optional)

INSTRUCTIONS

Preheat the oven to 400°F. Line a baking sheet with parchment paper.

In a large bowl, combine the eggplants, olive oil, and salt and toss to coat the eggplant in oil. The eggplant may absorb the oil and not become completely coated, but this is okay.

Spread the eggplant out in a single layer on the lined baking sheet.

Roast for 25 to 30 minutes, or until soft and golden brown on the edges.

In a small bowl, combine the oyster sauce, chili garlic sauce, and sugar. Transfer the roasted eggplant to a large bowl, pour the oyster sauce mixture over the top, and stir to combine. Add the cilantro leaves, if using, and stir to combine.

Serve warm as-is, or spooned over a bowl of hot rice.

Chef's Tip: Chili garlic sauce, sometimes called sambal, is a chunky paste made of crushed red peppers and garlic. It's intensely hot and flavorful, and goes great with meat, vegetables, and eggs. You can find this sauce in the Asian section of most grocery stores or at any Asian or Indian market.

Indian Skillet Potatoes

$

Potatoes have a reputation for being boring, but really they're just *waiting* for you to season them with anything your heart desires. This blend of Indian spices is warm, earthy, aromatic, and just a little spicy. The creamy potatoes provide the perfect backdrop and fresh cilantro adds a bright, fresh kick of flavor. If you're not a cilantro person, these potatoes are still delightful on their own. And if you prefer, use just a pinch of cayenne for less spicy potatoes, or leave it out completely for mild potatoes.

Serves 6

INGREDIENTS

3 pounds potatoes, cut into 1-inch cubes

2 teaspoons ground turmeric

1 teaspoon ground cumin

½ teaspoon ground cinnamon

⅛ teaspoon cayenne pepper

½ teaspoon salt

3 tablespoons vegetable oil

2 cloves garlic, minced

¼ bunch fresh cilantro, leaves only, roughly chopped (optional)

INSTRUCTIONS

Place the potatoes in a medium pot and add enough cool water to cover by 1 inch. Cover the pot and bring the water to a boil over high heat. Boil for about 5 minutes, or just until the potatoes can be pierced with a fork, but are not mushy or falling apart. Drain the potatoes in a colander.

In a small bowl, combine the turmeric, cumin, cinnamon, cayenne pepper, and salt. Set aside.

In a large skillet, heat the vegetable oil over medium heat. Add the garlic and cook for 1 to 2 minutes, or just until it begins to soften. Add the cooked potatoes and spice mix and sauté until the potatoes become slightly crispy on the edges, 7 to 10 minutes. Only stir the potatoes occasionally as they cook. Overstirring will prevent the surface of the potatoes from developing a nice brown, crispy layer.

Sprinkle the cilantro over the potatoes. Serve hot.

Lemon-Butter Green Beans $

Serves 4

This is my favorite side dish when I need something easy and green. The classic combination of lemon and butter is simple, bright, and works with just about any main dish. I've been making it for years because it's so quick, simple, and unbelievably delicious. Despite being one of the very first recipes that I ever posted to the blog, I had to include this recipe in the book so that *everyone* would know how to make this easy, classic side dish.

INGREDIENTS

1 pound green beans

1 medium lemon

2 tablespoons butter

Salt

Ground black pepper

INSTRUCTIONS

Snap the stems off of the green beans and then snap each bean into 1- to 2-inch pieces.

Place the green beans in a medium saucepan or skillet and add about 1 inch of water. Cover, set over high heat, and bring the water to a boil. Steam the beans for about 5 minutes, or until they are bright green and slightly tender. Drain the beans in a colander.

Using a Microplane or a small-holed cheese grater, scrape off the thin yellow layer of zest from the lemon (do not grate down to the white pith). Juice the lemon into a small bowl and set aside.

Add the lemon zest and butter to the pan in which you cooked the beans and set the pan over medium-low heat to melt the butter. Let the lemon zest simmer in the hot butter for 1 to 2 minutes.

Add the steamed green beans to the pan and toss them in the lemon butter to coat. Sprinkle the lemon juice over the beans and season with salt and pepper to taste.

Italian Spaghetti Squash $$

Serves 4

Spaghetti squash is not only healthy, but it's also super fun to eat. The flesh of this magical squash separates into perfect spaghetti-like strands once baked, making an excellent low-carb substitute for pasta. Most spaghetti squash recipes I've come across are laden with heavy cream sauces and cheese, but this version is lighter and still bursting with flavor. Spaghetti squash adopts the flavor of anything you add to it, so I've stuck with simple Italian herbs and spices and just a touch of Parmesan for depth. If you want a heartier meal, try adding a scoop of my Easy Meat Sauce (page 76) for a truly spaghetti-like experience.

INGREDIENTS

- 1 medium spaghetti squash (about 3 pounds)
- 2 tablespoons salted butter
- 1 tablespoon Italian seasoning blend
- 2 tablespoons grated Parmesan
- ¼ bunch fresh flat-leaf parsley, chopped
- Salt
- 2 Roma tomatoes, chopped

INSTRUCTIONS

Preheat the oven to 375°F.

Using the tip of a sharp knife or a heavy-duty fork, prick through the skin of the spaghetti squash several times on all sides. Place the squash in a large casserole dish and bake for 45 to 60 minutes, or until the flesh is fairly soft and gives in when squeezed. The exact cooking time will depend on the girth of your squash. Check it at 45 minutes and continue baking if it is not yet soft.

Remove the squash from the oven and set aside until cool enough to handle. Use a sharp knife to halve the squash lengthwise. Carefully scrape the seeds out with a spoon, trying not to scrape out the flesh in the process. Use a fork to scrape the squash flesh out of the skin and into a bowl. The flesh should separate into thin, spaghettilike strands all the way down to the thick skin.

Add the butter, Italian seasoning, Parmesan, and parsley to the squash. Stir to combine, allowing the residual heat from the squash to melt the butter. Season with salt to taste.

Either stir the tomatoes into the squash mixture or sprinkle them over the top before serving. The squash can be served in a bowl, or spooned back in its original skin for a more dramatic presentation.

 Chef's Tip: Italian seasoning blend is an easy way to add a burst of flavor to pasta, pizza, or sauces when you don't want to take the time to measure out several spices. Simply sprinkle it on for added flavor.

Firecracker Cauliflower $

Forget Flamin' Hot Cheetos—this cauliflower is where it's at! It's spicy, garlicky, salty, and will turn your fingertips red just like those spicy cheese poofs do—except it's made of *vegetables*! This spicy cauliflower is so good that I have a hard time not eating it raw, even before it goes in the oven. To dampen the flames, try serving with The "Real Deal" Chip Dip (page 68) or Lighter Ranch Dressing (page 72) for dipping.

Serves 3 to 4

INGREDIENTS

1 tablespoon paprika

¼ teaspoon garlic powder

¼ teaspoon cayenne pepper

½ teaspoon salt

Freshly cracked black pepper

1 large head cauliflower, cored and cut into bite-size florets

2 tablespoons olive oil

INSTRUCTIONS

Preheat the oven to 400°F. Line a rimmed baking sheet with foil and coat the foil with nonstick cooking spray.

In a small bowl, combine the paprika, garlic powder, cayenne pepper, salt, and some black pepper.

Place the cauliflower florets in a large bowl, drizzle them with the olive oil, and sprinkle the spice mix over the top. Toss the cauliflower until it is well coated in oil and spices. (The more you toss, the more the coating will spread, so be sure to toss well, but be gentle to avoid breaking up the florets.)

Spread the cauliflower in a single layer on the prepared baking sheet. Roast for 30 minutes, or until tender. Serve warm.

Chipotle–Sweet Potato Quesadillas $$

Serves 6

It's true, I love just about anything stuffed into a tortilla, but the way I feel about these quesadillas goes beyond love. There is so much flavor bursting out of every bite that it should almost be illegal. The filling is a little sweet, a little spicy, a little smoky, and super creamy all at the same time. If you like Southwestern flavors, you're sure to love these unique quesadillas.

INGREDIENTS

1 medium sweet potato (1½ to 2 pounds)

1 (15-ounce) can black beans, drained and rinsed

3 green onions, thinly sliced

¼ bunch fresh cilantro

1 (7-ounce) can chipotle peppers in adobo sauce

½ teaspoon ground cumin

1 cup shredded cheddar

6 large burrito-size flour tortillas

INSTRUCTIONS

Prick the sweet potato several times with a fork. Wrap it loosely in a paper towel and microwave on high for 5 minutes. Carefully squeeze the sweet potato to see if it is tender all the way through. If not, continue to microwave in 1-minute increments until it is soft. The potato will be very hot, so be careful! Set aside to cool while you prepare the rest of the filling.

In a large bowl, combine the black beans, green onions, and cilantro and toss.

Take 2 chipotle peppers from the can of adobo sauce and chop them finely. Add the chopped peppers and 2 teaspoons of the adobo sauce from the can to the bowl with the beans. Add the cumin and cheese and toss to combine.

When the sweet potato is cool enough to handle, scoop the flesh out of the skin with a spoon and add it to the bowl. Mix all the ingredients in the bowl until well combined.

Heat a skillet over medium heat. Place about ½ cup of sweet potato filling in each tortilla. Spread the filling over half of the tortilla and then fold the empty half over the top. Cook each tortilla in the skillet until golden and crispy on each side and the cheese is melted, about 5 minutes per side.

 Chef's Tip: Instead of using a microwave, you can bake the sweet potatoes ahead of time in an oven. Prick the skin of the potato as directed above and then bake in a preheated 400°F oven for 45 to 60 minutes, or until it is soft all the way through.

BUDGET BYTE Even though chipotle peppers in adobo sauce come in a very small can, I rarely use more than one pepper per recipe. The rest gets frozen in a small freezer bag for later use. You can also freeze them individually in an ice cube tray and then transfer them to a freezer bag for storage.

Ginger Snow Peas $$

Serves 4

This is a quick and simple stir-fry that makes a delicious side to any Asian-inspired meal. The mouthwatering combination of garlic and ginger is flavorful enough to add a punch, but not so strong that the subtle sweetness of the snow pea is lost. I like to use frozen snow peas because fresh can be quite pricey and are hard to find out of season. Frozen snow peas are also preblanched, which means they'll cook quicker. You can have this super-flavorful and fresh side dish ready to eat in under ten minutes.

INGREDIENTS

2 tablespoons vegetable oil

2 cloves garlic, minced

2-inch piece fresh ginger, peeled

1 (12-ounce) package frozen snow peas

1 teaspoon soy sauce, plus more
   as needed

INSTRUCTIONS

In a large skillet, heat the vegetable oil over medium heat. Add the garlic and, using a small-holed cheese grater or a Microplane, grate the ginger straight into the skillet. Sauté the garlic and ginger for 1 to 2 minutes, or until the garlic begins to soften.

Add the snow peas to the skillet and sauté until they are heated through, 5 to 7 minutes. Drizzle the soy sauce over the top and toss to coat. Taste the peas and add more soy sauce as needed. Serve hot.

Triple-Herb Mashed Potatoes

Is there anything more comforting than mashed potatoes? That warm mountain of starchy goodness with a pat of rich butter melting over top is difficult to resist. Mashed potatoes are filling, inexpensive, and can be flavored with a myriad of different seasonings. My favorite combination is a little bit of chicken broth and classic herbs, like garlic, thyme, oregano, and parsley. The herbs pack a huge flavor punch while the chicken broth provides depth without adding a lot of fat or calories. These potatoes have so much flavor that you won't even need to pile on the butter and cream.

Serves 4

INGREDIENTS

2 pounds potatoes

1 clove garlic, minced

2 tablespoons salted butter

½ cup chicken broth

2 tablespoons chopped fresh flat-leaf parsley

¼ teaspoon dried thyme

¼ teaspoon dried oregano

¼ teaspoon salt

Freshly cracked black pepper

INSTRUCTIONS

Peel the potatoes, if desired, and cut them into 1-inch cubes. Place the cubed potatoes in a medium pot and add enough cool water to cover by 1 inch. Bring the water to a boil over high heat and cook the potatoes for about 7 minutes, or until they are very tender and fall apart when pierced with a fork.

Drain the potatoes in a colander and return them to the warm pot with the heat turned off. Add the garlic to the potatoes along with the butter and chicken broth. Mash the potatoes to your desired consistency.

Add the parsley, thyme, oregano, salt, and some pepper to the potatoes. Stir until combined. Set aside, covered, for 5 minutes to allow the heat and steam to infuse the flavors. Taste and adjust the seasoning, if necessary.

Chef's Tip: This recipe can easily be made vegetarian by substituting vegetable broth for the chicken broth.

Roasted Carrots & Zucchini $

Food tastes better when it's pretty. That's just how it works. Vegetables in particular tend to suffer from the ugly duckling syndrome, but not these roasted carrot and zucchini sticks. Cutting the vegetables into matchsticks and combining their contrasting bright orange and green colors creates instant visual appeal. While their appearance may tempt you to have a first bite, their flavor is what will have you coming back for more. Roasting caramelizes the vegetables' natural sugars, creating a deep, subtle sweetness. A simple seasoning of salt, pepper, and thyme allows their natural flavors to shine through. Simple, flavorful, and good—the way food should be.

Serves 6

INGREDIENTS

1 pound carrots

1 medium zucchini

2 tablespoons olive oil

½ teaspoon dried thyme

½ teaspoon salt

Freshly cracked black pepper

INSTRUCTIONS

Preheat the oven to 400°F. Line a rimmed baking sheet with parchment paper or foil.

Cut the carrots and zucchini into ¼- to ½-inch-thick matchsticks, 3 to 4 inches long.

Place the vegetables in a large bowl and add the olive oil, thyme, salt, and pepper to taste. Toss to coat.

Spread the vegetables out in a single layer on the lined baking sheet. Roast for 30 minutes, or until soft and slightly golden brown on the edges. Serve hot.

Eleven

DESSERTS

My sweet tooth isn't big, but it *is* feisty! I don't get cravings often, but when I do they must be satisfied immediately. I like to make desserts that use pantry staples, so that I can whip them up on the fly. Whenever possible I try to work some fresh fruit into the splurge to reduce the post-dessert guilt. Plus, seasonal fruit is often much less expensive than butter, cream, or chocolate. Here are a few of my favorite sweet-tooth fixes for when you're having "one of those days."

Lemon-Raspberry Yogurt Cake   216

Microwave Apple Crumble for
One   218

Apricot-Walnut Bars   219

Strawberry–Cream Cheese
Quesadillas   220

"The One" Chocolate Mug Cake   221

Peach Bubble Cake   222

Apple Pie Bites   224

Monkey Bread   226

Chocolate-Cherry Biscotti   228

Chai-Spiced Almonds   230

Lemon-Raspberry Yogurt Cake $

Serves 8

I'm crazy about lemon, and when you combine it with a little sugar, vanilla, and creamy yogurt, you've got something that's absolutely to die for. Raspberries provide just the right sweet-tart contrast and add stunning red color. This dessert bread is perfect with an afternoon cup of coffee or tea, or any time that sweet tooth hits.

INGREDIENTS

2 cups all-purpose flour

½ teaspoon salt

1 tablespoon baking powder

1 medium lemon

¾ cup granulated sugar

¾ cup plain yogurt

2 large eggs

½ teaspoon vanilla extract

½ cup vegetable oil

1 cup fresh or frozen raspberries

1 cup powdered sugar

INSTRUCTIONS

Preheat the oven to 350°F. Coat a loaf pan with nonstick cooking spray.

In a medium bowl, stir together the flour, salt, and baking powder.

Using a Microplane or a small-holed cheese grater, scrape off the thin yellow layer of zest from the lemon (do not grate down to the white pith). Juice the lemon into a small bowl and set aside.

In a large bowl, combine the granulated sugar and lemon zest. Rub the sugar and zest together slightly with your hands to help release the zest's flavorful oil.

Add the yogurt, eggs, vanilla, oil, and half of the lemon juice (about 2 tablespoons) to the sugar mixture and whisk until smooth.

Pour the flour mixture into the yogurt mixture and gently stir until it forms a thick batter. Try not to overmix—it's okay if the batter is slightly lumpy. Gently fold in the raspberries (if using frozen raspberries, no thawing is needed).

Pour the batter into the prepared loaf pan. Bake for 55 minutes, or until the top is slightly golden brown and a toothpick inserted into the center comes out clean. After baking, run a knife around the edges of the loaf pan and gently turn the cake out onto a wire rack to cool.

To make the icing, in a small bowl, stir together the remaining lemon juice (about 2 tablespoons) and powdered sugar until smooth. (If you don't have 2 tablespoons of juice, use water to make up the difference.) The icing should be thick but smooth.

Allow the cake to cool completely, and then pour the icing over the top.

 Chef's Tip: Full- or low-fat yogurt works best for this recipe. Nonfat yogurt may give the cake a slightly rubbery texture.

Microwave Apple Crumble for One $

Serves 1

This super-simple "dessert in a cup" is the perfect quick fix when you need something naughty, but don't want to make a whole pie or dessert. Because this recipe uses just pantry staples, you can whip it up any time you have an extra apple lying around. Use the recipe below for one serving, or go ahead and double the recipe to use the whole apple and share with a friend!

FOR THE APPLE FILLING

½ medium apple, cut into bite-size pieces

1 teaspoon brown sugar

½ teaspoon cornstarch

⅛ teaspoon ground cinnamon

Pinch of ground cloves

Pinch of salt

FOR THE CRUMBLE TOPPING

½ tablespoon salted butter

1 tablespoon all-purpose flour

1½ tablespoons old-fashioned rolled oats

½ tablespoon brown sugar

INSTRUCTIONS

To make the apple filling, in a small bowl, combine the apple, brown sugar, cornstarch, cinnamon, cloves, and salt and toss to coat the apple pieces in the sugar and spices. Place the mixture in the bottom of a microwave-safe mug.

To make the crumble topping, in a small bowl, combine the butter, flour, oats, and brown sugar. Use your hands to rub the ingredients together until they form an even mixture that is slightly granular in texture. Sprinkle the mixture over the apple in the mug.

Microwave the mug on high for 90 seconds to 2 minutes, or until the apple is soft and gooey.

Apricot-Walnut Bars

I try so hard to be good, *so* hard. But sometimes I just need something sweet to nosh on. The subtle sweetness of the dried apricots, bananas, and a touch of brown sugar is just enough to quiet my sweet tooth, while oats and walnuts leave my belly full and my hunger squashed. Whether it's an after-dinner treat or a midmorning snack, these granola-like Apricot-Walnut Bars work double-duty as a dessert or mini meal. You can customize these bars to use whatever dried fruit or nuts you have on hand, but I'm partial to golden apricots and rich walnuts!

Serves 9

INGREDIENTS

1 cup mashed ripe bananas (2 to 3 medium bananas)

½ teaspoon vanilla extract

2 tablespoons brown sugar

½ teaspoon salt

⅓ cup chopped dried apricots

⅓ cup chopped walnuts

2 cups old-fashioned rolled oats

INGREDIENTS

Preheat the oven to 350°F. Line an 8-by-8-inch casserole dish with parchment paper.

In a medium bowl, combine the bananas, vanilla, brown sugar, and salt and stir to evenly combine.

Stir the apricots and walnuts into the banana mixture. Finally, stir in the oats.

Press the oat mixture evenly into the bottom of the prepared dish. Bake for 30 minutes, or until the edges are golden brown. Remove from the baking dish and set on a wire rack to cool, then cut into 9 equal bars, and enjoy.

Serves 3

You know how sometimes you want some cheesecake, but you don't want to make a *whole* cheesecake? (Who wants a *whole* cheesecake taunting them from the refrigerator all day and night? Not me.) These neat little quesadillas will give you your cheesecake fix without all the baking hassle and without a whole cake left over to haunt you in your sleep. Win-win. Just be careful—their ooey-gooey goodness can be messy!

INGREDIENTS

½ pound fresh or frozen strawberries

4 ounces cream cheese, at room temperature

¼ cup powdered sugar

¼ teaspoon vanilla extract

3 (8-inch) flour tortillas

INSTRUCTIONS

Thaw the strawberries, if frozen. Roughly chop the strawberries into small pieces.

In a small bowl, whisk together the cream cheese, powdered sugar, and vanilla.

Spread one-third of the cream cheese mixture over half of each tortilla. Sprinkle the strawberry pieces over the cream cheese and then fold the tortillas in half.

Lightly coat a medium skillet with nonstick cooking spray. Cook the quesadillas over medium heat until golden brown and crispy on each side. Allow to cool just slightly before eating, as the filling will be very hot.

"The One" Chocolate Mug Cake $

This little cup of heaven is just the right amount of *naughty* to make you feel *nice*. When you only need a few bites of something rich, you can whip this up in minutes without having to make a special trip to the store for ingredients. With just a few pantry staples, you're on your way to having a cup of rich, moist chocolate cake with a warm, gooey peanut butter center!

Serves 1

INGREDIENTS

2 tablespoons all-purpose flour

1 tablespoon unsweetened cocoa powder

1 tablespoon sugar

¼ teaspoon baking powder

Pinch of salt

2 tablespoons milk

1 tablespoon vegetable oil

1 tablespoon peanut butter

INSTRUCTIONS

In a microwave-safe coffee mug, combine the flour, cocoa powder, sugar, baking powder, and salt and stir to evenly combine.

Add the milk and vegetable oil and stir until a smooth, chocolatey batter forms. Push the peanut butter down into the center of the chocolate batter.

Microwave for 45 seconds on high power.

Enjoy!

Chef's Tip: For extra richness, add a few drops of vanilla extract or a few chocolate chips. The peanut butter can be substituted with other fillings like Nutella, jam, or caramel sauce.

Peach Bubble Cake $

Serves 8

This dessert can't figure out if it's a pie, cake, or cobbler, but I don't care because it's delicious. The bottom half is a gooey, cinnamon-flavored peach pie filling and the top half is a classic vanilla cake. The result looks something like a peach cobbler, but with a less biscuit-y topping. But let's stop trying to label it and just enjoy it for what it is.

FOR THE PEACH FILLING

1 pound fresh or frozen peach slices

¼ cup brown sugar

¼ teaspoon ground cinnamon

½ teaspoon cornstarch

2 tablespoons salted butter

FOR THE CAKE TOPPING

½ cup (1 stick) salted butter, at room temperature

1 cup granulated sugar

2 large eggs, at room temperature

1 teaspoon vanilla extract

1½ cups all-purpose flour

1½ teaspoons baking powder

½ cup milk

INSTRUCTIONS

Preheat the oven to 350°F.

To make the peach filling, place the peach slices in the bottom of a 9-inch pie dish or 8-by-8-inch casserole dish. In a small bowl, stir together the brown sugar, cinnamon, and cornstarch. Sprinkle the brown sugar mixture over the peaches and toss to coat. Cut the butter into small chunks and sprinkle it over the peaches. Bake the peaches for 30 minutes.

While the peaches are baking, prepare the cake topping: In a medium bowl, beat together the butter and granulated sugar until the mixture is light and creamy in texture, about 3 minutes. Add the eggs and vanilla and beat again until smooth.

In a separate small bowl, stir together the flour and baking powder. Slowly beat half of the flour mixture into the butter mixture, and then beat in half of the milk. Repeat with the remaining flour mixture and milk.

Briefly stir the peaches to redistribute the sugar and butter mixture. Pour the cake batter over the top, making sure to evenly cover all the peaches. Place the dish on a baking sheet to catch any filling that may bubble up and out while baking. Bake the cake for 35 minutes, or until the cake is golden brown on top and the peach filling is bubbling up around the edges.

Apple Pie Bites $

As if pie needs to be any more addictive, these cute little apple pie bites beg you to take one after another. They're super cute as a party appetizer, or perfect for when you just don't want to bake a whole pie. You can easily double the recipe to feed a crowd, or make it faster and easier by using store-bought pie dough.

INGREDIENTS

1 cup all-purpose flour

½ teaspoon granulated sugar

½ cup (1 stick) salted butter, cold

¼ cup ice water

2 tablespoons brown sugar

½ teaspoon ground cinnamon

⅛ teaspoon ground cloves

1 medium apple

INSTRUCTIONS

Combine the flour and granulated sugar in a large bowl and stir to evenly combine. Cut 7 tablespoons of the cold butter into chunks and add them to the flour mixture. (Reserve the remaining 1 tablespoon butter for the filling.) Use your hands or a pastry cutter to work the butter into the flour mixture until it becomes granular in texture, with only a few small pea-size pieces of butter visible.

Add the ice water and stir until the mixture begins to form a dough with no dry bits left on the bottom of the bowl. Form the dough into a ball, wrap it tightly in plastic wrap, and refrigerate for 30 minutes.

Preheat the oven to 350°F. Line a baking sheet with parchment paper.

Take the dough out of the refrigerator and roll it out into a disc 10 inches in diameter. If the edges crack when you roll out the dough, simply pinch them back together.

Place the reserved 1 tablespoon butter in a small bowl and microwave for 15 to 20 seconds, or just until melted. Add the brown sugar, cinnamon, and cloves to the butter and stir to combine. Spread the butter mixture thinly over the disc of pie dough. Cut the disc into 12 equal-size wedges.

Cut the apple into 12 equal-size wedges and remove the core. Place one apple wedge at the wide end of each pie dough triangle and roll up the dough like a crescent roll.

Place the wrapped apple wedges on the lined baking sheet. Bake for 35 minutes, or until the pie crust is slightly golden brown. Let the apple pie bites cool for 5 minutes before eating.

 Chef's Tip: It takes some practice to make these pretty, but believe me, no one will complain if you keep practicing!

Monkey Bread $

Serves 8

I have such fond memories of monkey bread from when I was little. Monkey bread elicited more excitement in our household than any other dessert. Can you imagine five kids all vying for a chance to get their fingers into one sticky loaf? It was complete chaos, but it was fun and very inexpensive. This recipe only uses pantry staples, which means you can make it with very little planning and for very little cash. I've provided a recipe for home-made dough below, but it can also be made with store-bought refrigerated bread dough if you're short on time.

FOR THE DOUGH

2 teaspoons active dry yeast

¾ cup warm water

3 tablespoons granulated sugar

2 tablespoons salted butter

1 large egg

1 teaspoon salt

2½ to 3 cups all-purpose flour

FOR THE TOPPING

¼ cup granulated sugar

½ tablespoon ground cinnamon

6 tablespoons salted butter

¼ cup brown sugar

½ teaspoon vanilla extract

INSTRUCTIONS

To make the dough, in a small bowl, combine the yeast, warm water, and granulated sugar and stir until the yeast has dissolved. Let stand for 5 minutes, or until the yeast becomes thick and frothy on top.

Microwave the butter in a small bowl for 15 to 20 seconds, or just until melted. Whisk the melted butter, egg, and salt into the yeast mixture.

In a large bowl, combine the yeast mixture and 1 cup of the flour and stir until the mixture is smooth.

Continue adding more flour to the bowl, ½ cup at a time, until you can no longer stir the mixture with a spoon. Turn the dough out onto a floured surface and knead it for 5 minutes, adding more flour as needed to keep it from sticking. (You may not need to use all 3½ cups of the flour.)

Shape the dough into a ball, place it back in the mixing bowl, cover it loosely with plastic, and allow it to rise for 1 hour, or until doubled in volume.

Punch the dough down to deflate it, place it on a clean work surface, and cut it into small, ½-inch pieces (about 32 pieces in total).

To make the topping, in a small bowl, combine the granulated sugar and cinnamon. Add a few pieces of dough at a time and toss them to coat in the sugar mixture. Place the coated dough pieces in a pie plate or Bundt pan coated with nonstick cooking spray. Sprinkle the remaining sugar mixture over the dough balls in the pan. Set aside to rise for 1 hour, or until doubled in volume.

Preheat the oven to 350°F.

In a microwave-safe bowl or small saucepan, melt the butter. Stir in the brown sugar and vanilla and pour the butter mixture over the coated dough balls in the pan.

Bake the bread for 30 minutes, or until golden brown on top. While the bread is still warm, turn it upside down onto a plate so that it comes out of its baking dish. Allow the bread to cool until it is easily handled with bare hands and then enjoy!

 Chef's Tip: If you're short on time, you can use store-bought refrigerated bread or biscuit dough in place of the homemade bread dough.

Chocolate-Cherry Biscotti $

Makes 30

I absolutely adore a really good biscotti: crisp enough to hold up to being dipped in a piping-hot cup of coffee, but not so rock hard that they'll cut open the roof of my mouth. This rich combination of cocoa and dried cherries pairs perfectly with the earthy flavor of coffee. Can't find dried cherries? No problem! Substitute chocolate chips or dried cranberries for an equally delicious biscotti!

INGREDIENTS

1½ cups all-purpose flour

⅓ cup unsweetened cocoa powder

1 teaspoon baking powder

¼ teaspoon salt

4 tablespoons salted butter, room temperature

2 large eggs

1 cup sugar

1 teaspoon vanilla extract

½ cup dried cherries

INSTRUCTIONS

Preheat the oven to 350°F. Line a baking sheet with parchment paper.

In a medium bowl, combine the flour, cocoa powder, baking powder, and salt and stir to evenly combine.

In a large bowl, whisk together the butter, eggs, sugar, and vanilla until light and creamy. (You can use a mixer for this step if you have one.) Stir in the dried cherries.

Add the flour mixture to the butter mixture and stir until a soft dough forms.

Divide the dough in half and form it into 2 flattened logs, about 3 inches wide and 8 inches long. Place the logs on the lined baking sheet. Bake for 35 minutes.

Remove the biscotti from the oven and allow to cool for about 5 minutes. Carefully transfer the baked biscotti logs to a cutting board and use a large, sharp knife to slice the logs crosswise on an angle into strips about ¾ inch wide. The biscotti will be delicate at this stage, so cut carefully. Lay the sliced biscotti back on the baking sheet and bake for 5 to 7 minutes more. Flip each biscotti over and bake for an additional 5 to 7 minutes on the other side.

Allow the biscotti to cool and then store in an airtight container at room temperature for up to 1 week. Extra biscotti can be frozen in an airtight zip-top freezer bag for up to six months. Simply thaw at room temperature before serving.

Chai-Spiced Almonds $$$

Makes
1 pound

Nuts are pretty expensive, but the price jumps even higher when they're roasted and candy coated. I know, I know, that scent that wafts to you from the mall kiosk is *really* hard to resist, but if you can just wait until you get home, you can make your whole house smell that good and enjoy the results at a fraction of the cost. You can use any type of nut and any blend of spices you want, but this recipe for chai-spiced almonds is my favorite. Have fun with it and make them your own!

INGREDIENTS

⅓ cup brown sugar

⅓ cup granulated sugar

1 teaspoon ground cinnamon

½ teaspoon ground ginger

¼ teaspoon ground cloves

¼ teaspoon ground cardamom (optional)

½ teaspoon salt

1 large egg

½ teaspoon vanilla extract

1 pound whole raw almonds

INSTRUCTIONS

Preheat the oven to 300°F. Line a baking sheet with parchment paper.

In a medium bowl, combine the brown sugar, granulated sugar, cinnamon, ginger, cloves, cardamom, if using, and salt. Stir until well combined.

Separate the egg white from the yolk and place the egg white in a large glass or metal bowl. Whisk the egg white until it is light and frothy, but not yet forming peaks. Add the vanilla and whisk briefly to combine.

Pour the nuts into the egg white mixture and stir to coat. Add the sugar and spices to the nuts and stir to coat again.

Pour the coated nuts on the lined baking sheet and spread them into a single layer. Bake for 30 minutes, stirring halfway through. Allow the nuts to cool before eating so that the candy coating can harden.

APPENDIX A: SAMPLE MENUS

Figuring out which recipes to serve together is a skill that gets easier with time. A well-rounded meal will have a variety of complementary flavors, colors, and textures, and have a good balance between proteins, carbohydrates, and vegetables. Another goal that I try to achieve with meal planning is combining recipes that share ingredients to reduce leftover or wasted ingredients.

These menu pairings will help get you accustomed to pairing flavors and textures, as well as make full use of the recipes in this book. For a meal-planning kick-start, begin here.

BEEF MENUS

Farmer Joes (page 142)
Tomato-Cheddar Soup (page 122)

- - -

Chili-Cheese Beef 'n' Mac (page 146)
Jalapeño Cornbread (page 45)

- - -

Beef & Bean Taquitos (page 150)
Creamy Cilantro-Lime Dressing (page 71)
Cumin-Lime Sweet Potato Sticks (page 198)

CHICKEN MENUS

Teriyaki Chicken Sliders (page 162)

Easy Asian Slaw (page 90)

- - -

Rosemary-Garlic Roasted Chicken & Potatoes (page 160)

Lemon-Butter Green Beans (page 204)

Soft 'n' Sweet Dinner Rolls (page 52)

- - -

Chicken Tamale Pie (page 158)

Cilantro-Lime Rice (page 182)

- - -

Coconut Chicken Curry (page 154)

Spiced Chickpeas (page 185)

PORK MENUS

Pasta e Fagioli (page 128)

Parmesan-Herb Drop Biscuits (page 43)

- - -

Pork with Balsamic-Cranberry Sauce (page 169)

Triple-Herb Mashed Potatoes (page 211)

Apple Dijon Kale Salad (page 87)

- - -

Chorizo–Sweet Potato Enchiladas (page 164)

Cilantro-Lime Rice (page 182)

Quick Chipotle Black Beans (page 184)

Herb-Roasted Pork Loin (page 167)

Tuscan White Beans (page 192)

Roasted Carrots & Zucchini (page 213)

- - -

Five-Spice Chops (page 166)

Pineapple Fried Rice (page 183)

Ginger Snow Peas (page 210)

- - -

One-Skillet Lasagna (page 111)

Super-Crunch Salad (page 80)

Italian Breadsticks (page 58)

SEAFOOD MENUS

Thai Steamed Fish (page 177)

Savory Coconut Rice (page 181)

Ginger Snow Peas (page 210)

- - -

Teriyaki Salmon with Sriracha Mayo (page 173)

Emerald Rice Salad (page 195)

- - -

Lemon-Garlic Shrimp Pasta (page 175)

Balsamic Tomato Bruschetta (page 69)

VEGETARIAN MENUS

Greek Chopped Salad (page 93)

Basic Hummus (page 62)

Naan (page 56)

– – –

Southwest Veggie & Rice Casserole (page 190)

Jalapeño Cornbread (page 45)

Cumin-Lime Sweet Potato Sticks (page 198)

– – –

Hearty Vegetable & Barley Soup (page 136)

Cheddar-Beer Bread (page 47)

– – –

Autumn Lentil Pilaf (page 186)

Carrot–Sweet Potato Soup (page 124)

Multigrain Rolls (page 54)

– – –

Chipotle–Sweet Potato Quesadillas (page 208)

Quick Chipotle Black Beans (page 184)

– – –

Zucchini-Pasta Bake (page 116)

Italian Breadsticks (page 58)

APPENDIX B:
VEGETARIAN & VEGAN RECIPES

Vegetarian Recipes

Apple-Cinnamon French Toast Casserole   *35*

Apple Pie Bites   *224*

Autumn Delight Baked Oatmeal   *20*

Avocado-Egg Toast   *30*

Banana Bread Baked Oatmeal   *18*

Banana-Nut Muffins   *31*

Breakfast Parfaits   *22*

Chai-Spiced Almonds   *230*

Cheddar-Beer Bread   *47*

Chipotle–Sweet Potato Quesadillas   *208*

Chocolate-Cherry Biscotti   *228*

Creamy Balsamic Dressing   *73*

Creamy Cilantro-Lime Dressing   *71*

Creamy Orzo with Spinach   *106*

Dijon Potato & Green Bean Salad   *94*

Easy Pad Thai   *112*

Garlic-Herb Pasta   *108*

Greek Chopped Salad   *93*

Honey-Wheat Biscuits   *41*

Honey-Wheat Sandwich Bread   *50*

Huevos Rancheros Bowls   *29*

Iced Orange-Cranberry Scones   33

Italian Baked Eggs   26

Italian Spaghetti Squash   205

Jalapeño Cornbread   45

Lemon-Butter Green Beans   204

Lemon-Parmesan Pasta with Peas   115

Lemon-Raspberry Yogurt Cake   216

Lentil & Feta Salad   83

Lighter Ranch Dressing   72

Microwave Apple Crumble for One   218

Monkey Bread   226

Naan   56

Parmesan-Herb Drop Biscuits   43

Peach Bubble Cake   222

Roasted Eggplant Pasta   102

Sesame-Ginger Dressing   74

Sesame Noodles   114

Soft 'n' Sweet Dinner Rolls   52

Southwest Veggie & Rice Casserole   190

Spinach & Artichoke Pasta   100

Strawberry–Cream Cheese Quesadillas   220

"The One" Chocolate Mug Cake   221

The "Real Deal" Chip Dip   68

Vinaigrette Slaw with Feta   86

Zucchini-Pasta Bake   116

Vegan Recipes

Apricot-Walnut Bars   219

Autumn Lentil Pilaf   186

Balsamic Tomato Bruschetta   69

Basic Hummus   62

Best Bean Dip   66

Cranberry-Almond Granola   24

Cumin, Lime & Chickpea Salad   85

Cumin-Lime Sweet Potato Sticks   198

Easy Asian Slaw   90

Emerald Rice Salad   195

Firecracker Cauliflower   207

Ginger Snow Peas   210

Hearty Vegetable & Barley Soup   136

Indian Skillet Potatoes   203

Italian Breadsticks   58

Mango, Jalapeño & Quinoa Salad   91

Multigrain Rolls   54

No-Knead Focaccia   48

Quick Chipotle Black Beans   184

Quick Salsa   64

Red Enchilada Sauce   77

Roasted Broccoli with Crispy Garlic   199

Roasted Carrots & Zucchini   213

Savory Coconut Rice   181

Spiced Chickpeas   185

Summer Melon Salad   82

Super-Crunch Salad   80

Taco Rice   180

Tomato & White Bean Salad   89

Tuscan White Beans   192

APPENDIX C:
VOLUME CONVERSIONS

- - - - - - - - - - - - - - - - - - -

One Gallon Equals:

3.8 liters

4 quarts

16 cups

128 fluid ounces

One Quart Equals:

.95 Liters

2 pints

4 cups

32 fluid ounces

One Cup Equals:

8 fluid ounces

16 tablespoons

237 milliliters

½ Cup Equals:

4 fluid ounces

8 tablespoons

24 teaspoons

118 milliliters

¼ Cup Equals:

2 fluid ounces

4 tablespoons

12 teaspoons

59 milliliters

One Tablespoon Equals:

½ fluid ounce

3 teaspoons

15 milliliters

ACKNOWLEDGMENTS

- -

A BIG Thank You to . . .

My excellent group of recipe testers, whose opinions were incredibly valuable: Andrea Anderson, Laura Bresnahan Laura Carscaddon, Roberto Cases, Emily Drew, Jessica Fisher, Erica Foulser, Sarah Groves, Jim Jorgensen, Monica Mark, Lindsay Parsons, Carrie Robinson, Rabia Shahid, and Emily Wunderlich.

My wonderful editor, Gigi Campo, and superstar agent, Sharon Bowers, for guiding me through this amazing experience and helping me make one of my lifelong dreams come true.

All of my friends, my family, and my coworkers at Tulane Medical Center for putting up with me during one of the most stressful years of my life! I love you guys!

And, as always, thank you to my amazing blog readers, who inspire me daily, teach me new things at every turn, and always bring a smile to my face. I can never thank you enough!

INDEX

$ (Bread 'n' Butter recipes), 4, 5
$$ (Frugal Foodie recipes), 4, 5
$$$ (Sensible Splurges recipes), 4, 5
❄ (Freezer-Friendly recipes), 5

active dry yeast, 39, 49
almonds
    Chai-Spiced Almonds, 230
    Cranberry-Almond Granola, 24–25
apples
    Apple-Cinnamon French Toast
        Casserole, 35–36
    Apple Dijon Kale Salad, 87–88
    Apple Pie Bites, 224–25
    Microwave Apple Crumble for
        One, 218
Apple-Cinnamon French Toast
    Casserole, 35–36
Apricot-Walnut Bars, 219
Artichoke & Spinach Pasta, 100–101
Asian-inspired dishes
    Asian Pork Lettuce Wraps, 171–72
    Easy Asian Slaw, 90
Asian markets, 112, 121, 153, 166,
    177, 181, 201, 202
Autumn-inspired dishes
    Autumn Delight Baked Oatmeal,
        20–21
    Autumn Lentil Pilaf, 186–87
avocados
    Avocado-Egg Toast, 30
    tips, 30, 195

baby spinach tip, 81
bacon
    grease from, 189, 194
    tips, 129
    White Beans with Spinach &
        Bacon, 188–89

Baked Eggs, Italian, 26
baked oatmeal
    Autumn Delight Baked Oatmeal,
        20–21
    Banana Bread Baked Oatmeal,
        18–19
bakeware, 9, 10
balsamic vinegar
    Balsamic Tomato Bruschetta, 69–70
    Creamy Balsamic Dressing, 73, 80
    Pork with Balsamic-Cranberry
        Sauce, 169–70
bananas
    Banana Bread Baked Oatmeal,
        18–19
    Banana-Nut Muffins, 31–32
    tips, 19, 32
Barley
    Hearty Vegetable & Barley
        Soup, 136–37
Bars, Apricot-Walnut, 219
Basic Hummus, 62–63
basil and salads, 89
beans
    Basic Hummus, 62–63
    Beef & Bean Taquitos, 71, 150–51
    Best Bean Dip, 66–67
    Calico Beans, 193–94
    Cumin, Lime & Chickpea
        Salad, 71, 85
    Dijon Potato & Green Bean
        Salad, 94–95
    Green Onion & Parsley
        Hummus, 62–63
    Jalapeño-Cilantro Hummus, 62–63
    Lemon-Butter Green Beans, 204
    Quick Chipotle Black Beans, 184
    Roasted Red Pepper Hummus,
        62–63

Spiced Chickpeas, 185
Tomato & White Bean Salad, 89
Tuscan White Beans, 192
White Beans with Spinach &
    Bacon, 188–89
Zesty Black Bean Soup, 139–40
See also rice, beans & lentils
beef
    Beef & Bean Taquitos, 71, 150–51
    Chili-Cheese Beef 'n' Mac, 146–47
    Farmer Joes, 142–43
    freezing beef tip, 151
    Ginger Beef 'n' Broccoli, 144–45
    Greek Steak Tacos, 148–49
    menus, 231
    Spicy Beef 'n' Noodles, 152–53
beef bouillon, 147
Beer-Bread, Cheddar, 37, 47
Best Bean Dip, 66–67
Better-Than-Mom's Chili, 134–35
Biscotti, Chocolate-Cherry, 228–29
biscuits
    Honey-Wheat Biscuits, 37, 41–42
    Parmesan-Herb Drop Biscuits, 37,
        43–44
    tip, 42
black beans
    Quick Chipotle Black Beans, 184
    Zesty Black Bean Soup, 139–40
blending hot soups tip, 140
blog, Budget Bytes, 3
bowls (Huevos Rancheros), preparing
    ahead of time, 29
bread machine yeast, 39
Bread 'n' Butter recipes ($), 4, 5
breads, 37–59
    active dry yeast, 39, 49
    bread machine yeast, 39
    cake yeast, 39

Cheddar-Beer Bread, 37, 47
Corn Muffins, 45–46
cutting bread tip, 51
freezing breads tips, 42, 51, 55, 57
fresh yeast, 39
Honey-Wheat Biscuits, 37, 41–42
Honey-Wheat Sandwich Bread,
    37, 50–51
instant yeast, 39, 49
Italian Breadsticks, 37, 58–59
Jalapeño Cornbread, 37, 45–46
kneading dough, 38, 40
Monkey Bread, 226–27
Multigrain Rolls, 37, 54–55, 132
Naan, 37, 56–57, 124
No-Knead Focaccia, 37, 48–49
Parmesan-Herb Drop Biscuits, 37,
    43–44
proofing (letting dough rise), 39, 40
quick breads, 37, 38
rapid-rise yeast, 39
Soft 'n' Sweet Dinner Rolls, 37,
    52–53
yeast breads, 37, 38–40
yeasts, 38–39, 49
See also Budget Bytes
Breadsticks, Italian, 37, 58–59
breakfast, 17–36
    Apple-Cinnamon French Toast
        Casserole, 35–36
    Autumn Delight Baked Oatmeal,
        20–21
    Avocado-Egg Toast, 30
    Banana Bread Baked Oatmeal,
        18–19
    Banana-Nut Muffins, 31–32
    Breakfast Parfaits, 22–23
    Cranberry-Almond Granola, 24–25
    Ham & Swiss Crustless Quiche,
        27–28
    Huevos Rancheros Bowls, 29
    Iced Orange-Cranberry Scones,
        33–34
    Italian Baked Eggs, 26
    See also Budget Bytes
broccoli
    Broccoli & Cheddar Soup, 132–33
    Ginger Beef 'n' Broccoli, 144–45
    Roasted Broccoli with Crispy
        Garlic, 199–200
    tips, 133, 145, 200
broth, 77, 123, 125, 147, 180, 212
brown lentils, 84, 127, 187
Bruschetta, Balsamic Tomato, 69–70
Bubble Cake, Peach, 222–23
Budget Bytes, 1–15

blog, 3
Bread 'n' Butter recipes ($), 4, 5
cooking adventure, 2, 3, 6
Freezer-Friendly recipes (❄), 5
Frugal Foodie recipes ($$), 4, 5
ingredients, 5, 6, 7–8
learning from failures, 6
measuring ingredients, 6
menus, 5–6, 231–34
Newbies Tips, 6
preheating your oven, 6
reading recipes before
    beginning, 6
Sensible Splurges recipes ($$$), 4, 5
volume conversions, 238
See also breads; breakfast; budget
    bytes tips; chef's tips; desserts;
    dressings, dips & sauces; kitchen
    basics; meat, poultry & seafood;
    pasta; rice, beans & lentils;
    salads; soups; vegan recipes;
    vegetables; vegetarian recipes
budget bytes tips
    baby spinach, 81
    bacon, 129, 189
    barley, 137
    beef, freezing, 151
    beef bouillon, 147
    biscuits, 42
    breads, freezing, 42, 51, 55, 57
    broccoli, 133, 200
    broth, 147
    bulk bins, 19, 25, 92, 137
    cabbage, 81, 86
    cheese, freezing, 117
    cherry tomatoes, 110
    chicken breasts, 97
    chicken broth (white wine
        substitute), 101
    chili garlic sauce (sambal), 202
    Chinese five-spice powder, 166
    chipotle peppers, 184, 209
    cream cheese (goat cheese
        substitute), 107
    curry powder, 131
    enchilada sauce, 105
    fettuccine noodles (lo mein noodles
        substitute), 153
    ginger, 75
    goat cheese ("chèvre") substitute
        (cream cheese), 107
    granola, 25
    lime juice, 85
    linguine (pad thai substitute), 113
    lo mein noodles substitute
        (fettuccine noodles), 153

mangoes substitute (pineapple), 92
mayonnaise, 68
meat thermometers, 168
melons, 82
oats, 19
pad thai substitute (linguine), 113
pasta, freezing, 117
pearled barley, 137
pineapple juice (leftover),
    23, 195
pineapple (mangoes substitute), 92
pork loin vs. pork tenderloin, 168
quinoa, 92
ramen noodles, 121
refrigerated salads, 88
rice vinegar, 75
rolls, 55
shredded cheese, 117
smoothies, 23, 81, 195
spices, 155
spinach, 81, 189
tahini, 75
toasted sesame oil, 75
tomatoes, 89, 110
tomato paste, 194
tuna, 110
vegetable juice, 135
white wine substitute (chicken
    broth), 101
See also Budget Bytes; chef's tips
Budget Byting Principles, 4, 5, 7–9
bulk bins, 19, 25, 92, 137
butter (cutting into flour) tip, 34

cabbage tips, 81, 86
cakes
    Lemon-Raspberry Yogurt
        Cake, 216–17
    "One, The" Chocolate Mug Cake,
        221
    Peach Bubble Cake, 222–23
cake yeast, 39
Calico Beans, 193–94
caramel sauce (peanut butter
    substitute), 221
carrots
    Carrot–Sweet Potato Soup, 124–25
    Roasted Carrots & Zucchini, 213
casseroles
    Apple-Cinnamon French Toast
        Casserole, 35–36
    Southwest Veggie & Rice Casserole,
        180, 190–91
Cauliflower, Firecracker, 72, 207
cayenne pepper tips, 155, 159
ceramic equipment, 9

Chai-Spiced Almonds, 230
cheddar cheese
    Broccoli & Cheddar Soup, 132–33
    Cheddar-Beer Bread, 37, 47
    Chili-Cheese Beef 'n' Mac, 146–47
    Tomato-Cheddar Soup, 122–23
cheese
    Broccoli & Cheddar Soup, 132–33
    Cheddar-Beer Bread, 37, 47
    Chili-Cheese Beef 'n' Mac, 146–47
    freezing cheese tip, 117
    Ham & Swiss Crustless Quiche,
        27–28
    Lemon-Parmesan Pasta with
        Peas, 115
    Lentil & Feta Salad, 83–84
    Parmesan-Herb Drop Biscuits, 37,
        43–44
    shredded cheese tip, 117
    Tomato-Cheddar Soup, 122–23
    Vinaigrette Slaw with Feta, 86
Chef's tips
    avocados, 30, 195
    bacon, cooking, 129
    bananas, 19, 32
    basil and salads, 89
    bean dip, 67
    beer bread, 47
    blending hot soups, 140
    bowls (Huevos Rancheros),
        preparing ahead of time, 29
    broccoli, 145, 200
    broth, 77, 123, 125, 180, 212
    brown lentils, 84, 127, 187
    butter (cutting into flour), 34
    cabbage, 86
    caramel sauce (peanut butter
        substitute), 221
    cayenne pepper, 155, 159
    chicken broth, 77, 180
    chicken broth substitute (vegetable
        broth), 123, 125, 212
    chiles, 66, 191
    chocolate in chili, 135
    chorizo, 165
    coarse sugar (icing substitute), 34
    corn muffins, 45–46
    curry powder, 155
    cutting bread, 51
    deli meat, 28
    eggplant, 103
    fat, importance to texture and
        flavor, 72, 73
    flank steak, 149
    focaccia toppings, 49
    French lentils, 84, 187

fry bread, 57
glossy, golden-brown rolls, 55
grease from meat, 189, 194
Greek yogurt (sour cream
    substitute), 68
green lentils, 84, 127, 187
herbs, 44
icing substitute (coarse sugar), 34
instant yeast vs. active dry yeast, 49
Italian seasoning blend, 206
jam (peanut butter substitute), 221
jasmine rice substitute (long-grain
    white rice), 172
lentils, 84, 127, 187
lime juice, 71, 113
long-grain white rice (jasmine rice
    substitute), 172
marinade, 161
Mason jars for parfaits, 22
mayonnaise, 73
meat, slicing, 170
meatballs, 157
Mexican chorizo vs. Spanish
    chorizo, 165
Nutella (peanut butter substitute),
    221
old-fashioned rolled oats vs. quick-
    cooking oats, 19
orange lentils, 84, 127
parfaits, 22
peanut butter substitute (Nutella,
    jam, caramel sauce), 221
poblano peppers, 165
pumpkin puree, 21
red lentils, 84, 127, 187
refrigerated bread/biscuit
    dough, 227
rice, 172
rice cooker, 181
rolls, 55
salads, customizing, 90
slicing meat, 170
soups, extra smooth, 123
soups (hot), blending, 140
sour cream substitute (Greek
    yogurt), 68
spinach, 107
sriracha mayo ("rooster
    sauce"), 174
sweet potatoes, 209
tahini, 63
thyme, 95
tomatoes, 66, 191
vanilla extract, 221
vegetable broth (chicken broth
    substitute), 123, 125, 212

vegetables, using extra, 121
yeast, 49
yellow lentils, 84, 127, 187
yogurt, 217
See also Budget Bytes; budget bytes
    tips
cherry tomatoes tip, 110
chèvre (goat cheese) substitute (cream
    cheese), 107
chicken
    chicken breasts tip, 97
    Chicken Tamale Pie, 158–59
    Chinese Chicken Noodle Soup,
        120–21
    Coconut Chicken Curry,
        154–55
    menus, 232
    Rosemary-Garlic Roasted Chicken
        & Potatoes, 160–61
    Southwest Chicken Salad,
        96–97
    Teriyaki Chicken Sliders, 90,
        162–63
chicken broth
    substitute (vegetable broth), 123,
        125, 212
    tips, 77, 180
    white wine substitute, 101
chickpeas
    Basic Hummus, 62–63
    Cumin, Lime & Chickpea Salad,
        71, 85
    Green Onion & Parsley Hummus,
        62–63
    Jalapeño-Cilantro Hummus,
        62–63
    Roasted Red Pepper Hummus,
        62–63
    Spiced Chickpeas, 185
chiles tips, 66, 191
chili
    Better-Than-Mom's Chili, 134–35
    Chili-Cheese Beef 'n' Mac, 146–47
chili garlic sauce (sambal), 202
chilling food before freezing, 12–13
Chinese Chicken Noodle Soup,
    120–21
Chinese five-spice powder, 166
Chip Dip ("Real Deal"), The, 68, 207
chipotle peppers
    Chipotle–Sweet Potato Quesadillas,
        208–9
    Quick Chipotle Black Beans, 184
    tips, 184, 209
chocolate
    chili, chocolate in, 135

Chocolate-Cherry Biscotti, 228–29
"One, The" Chocolate Mug Cake,
    221
Chopped Salad, Greek, 93
Chorizo & Sweet Potato Enchiladas,
    164–65
cilantro
    Cilantro-Lime Rice, 182
    Creamy Cilantro-Lime Dressing,
        71, 85, 150
    Jalapeño-Cilantro Hummus, 62–63
coarse sugar (icing substitute), 34
coconut
    Coconut Chicken Curry, 154–55
    Savory Coconut Rice, 181
community-supported agriculture
    (CSAs), 8–9
conversions, volume, 238
cooking adventure, 2, 3, 6
    See also Budget Bytes
Cornbread, Jalapeño, 37, 45–46
corn muffins, 45–46
cranberries
    Cranberry-Almond Granola, 24–25
    Iced Orange-Cranberry Scones,
        33–34
    Pork with Balsamic-Cranberry
        Sauce, 169–70
cream cheese (goat cheese
    substitute), 107
Creamy Balsamic Dressing, 73, 80
Creamy Cilantro-Lime Dressing, 71,
    85, 150
Creamy Orzo with Spinach, 106–7
Crumble for One, Microwave
    Apple, 218
Crustless Quiche, Ham & Swiss,
    27–28
CSAs (community-supported
    agriculture), 8–9
cumin
    Cumin, Lime & Chickpea Salad,
        71, 85
    Cumin-Lime Sweet Potato Sticks,
        71, 198
curry
    Coconut Chicken Curry, 154–55
    Curried Potato & Pea Soup,
        130–31
    tips, 131, 155
cutting bread tip, 51

deli meat tip, 28
desserts, 215–30
    Apple Pie Bites, 224–25
    Apricot-Walnut Bars, 219

Chai-Spiced Almonds, 230
Chocolate-Cherry Biscotti, 228–29
fruit in, 215
Lemon-Raspberry Yogurt Cake,
    216–17
Microwave Apple Crumble for
    One, 218
Monkey Bread, 226–27
"One, The" Chocolate Mug Cake,
    221
Peach Bubble Cake, 222–23
Strawberry–Cream Cheese
    Quesadillas, 220
    See also Budget Bytes
dijon
    Apple Dijon Kale Salad, 87–88
    Dijon Potato & Green Bean Salad,
        94–95
Dinner Rolls, Soft 'n' Sweet, 37,
    52–53
dips. See dressings, dips & sauces
dividing food before freezing, 12
dressings, dips & sauces, 61–77
    Balsamic Tomato Bruschetta, 69–70
    Basic Hummus, 62–63
    Best Bean Dip, 66–67
    Creamy Balsamic Dressing, 73, 80
    Creamy Cilantro-Lime Dressing,
        71, 85, 150
    Easy Meat Sauce, 76, 205
    Green Onion & Parsley Hummus,
        62–63
    Jalapeño-Cilantro Hummus, 62–63
    Lighter Ranch Dressing, 72, 207
    Quick Salsa, 64–65
    "Real Deal" Chip Dip, The, 68, 207
    Red Enchilada Sauce, 77, 104, 105
    Roasted Red Pepper Hummus,
        62–63
    Sesame-Ginger Dressing, 74–75
    See also Budget Bytes
Drop Biscuits, Parmesan-Herb, 37,
    43–44
dry goods, pantry staples, 11

Easy Asian Slaw, 90
Easy Meat Sauce, 76, 205
Easy Pad Thai, 112–13
eggplant
    Roasted Eggplant Pasta, 102–3
    Spicy Roasted Eggplant, 201–2
    tip, 103
eggs
    Avocado-Egg Toast, 30
    Huevos Rancheros Bowls, 29
    Italian Baked Eggs, 26

Emerald Rice Salad, 195
enchiladas
    Chorizo–Sweet Potato Enchiladas,
        164–65
    Loaded Enchilada Pasta, 77, 104–5
Enchilada Sauce, Red, 77, 104, 105
equipment, kitchen basics, 9–11
ethnic markets, 8, 131, 153, 155, 166

Facebook, 2
failures, learning from, 6
Farmer Joes, 142–43
farmer's markets, 8–9
fat, importance to texture and flavor,
    72, 73
feta cheese
    Lentil & Feta Salad, 83–84
    Vinaigrette Slaw with Feta, 86
fettuccine noodles (lo mein noodles
    substitute), 153
Firecracker Cauliflower, 72, 207
fish
    Pasta with Tuna & Olives, 109–10
    Thai Steamed Fish, 177–78
Five-Spice Chops, 166, 181
flank steak tip, 149
flatbread (Naan), 37, 56–57, 124
Focaccia, No-Knead, 37, 48–49
food budgets, 1–2
    See also Budget Bytes
Freezer-Friendly recipes (✲), 5
freezing breads tips, 42, 51, 55, 57
freezing food, 5, 8, 12–15
French lentils, 84, 187
French Toast Casserole,
    Apple-Cinnamon, 35–36
fresh yeast, 39
Fried Rice, Pineapple, 183
Frugal Foodie recipes ($$), 4, 5
fruit
    desserts and, 215
    See also specific fruit
fry bread, 57

garlic
    Garlic-Herb Pasta, 108
    Lemon-Garlic Shrimp Pasta,
        175–76
    Roasted Broccoli with Crispy
        Garlic, 199–200
    Rosemary-Garlic Roasted Chicken
        & Potatoes, 160–61
ginger
    Ginger Snow Peas, 210
    Sesame-Ginger Dressing, 74–75
    tip, 75

glass equipment, 9
glossy, golden-brown rolls, 55
gluten and yeast breads, 38
goat cheese ("chèvre") substitute
    (cream cheese), 107
"grab 'n' go" lunches, 8
Granola, Cranberry-Almond, 24–25
grease from meat, 189, 194
Greek-inspired dishes
    Greek Chopped Salad, 93
    Greek Lemon & Orzo Soup, 138
    Greek Steak Tacos, 148–49
Greek yogurt (sour cream
    substitute), 68
green beans
    Dijon Potato & Green Bean Salad,
        94–95
    Lemon-Butter Green Beans, 204
green lentils, 84, 127, 187
Green Onion & Parsley Hummus,
    62–63

Ham & Swiss Crustless Quiche,
    27–28
Hearty Vegetable & Barley Soup,
    136–37
herbs
    Garlic-Herb Pasta, 108
    Herb-Roasted Pork Loin, 167–68
    Parmesan-Herb Drop Biscuits,
        37, 43–44
    tip, 44
    Triple-Herb Mashed Potatoes,
        211–12
honey
    Honey-Wheat Biscuits, 37, 41–42
    Honey-Wheat Sandwich Bread,
        37, 50–51
household budgets, 1
    See also Budget Bytes
How to Stock a Kitchen, 5, 9–11
Huevos Rancheros Bowls, 29
hummus
    Basic Hummus, 62–63
    Green Onion & Parsley Hummus,
        62–63
    Jalapeño-Cilantro Hummus, 62–63
    Roasted Red Pepper Hummus,
        62–63

Iced Orange-Cranberry Scones,
    33–34
icing substitute (coarse sugar), 34
Indian Skillet Potatoes, 203
ingredients, using wisely, 5, 6, 7–8
instant yeast, 39, 49

Italian-inspired dishes
    Italian Baked Eggs, 26
    Italian Breadsticks, 37, 58–59
    Italian Spaghetti Squash, 205–6
Italian sausage
    Easy Meat Sauce, 76, 205
    Lentil & Sausage Stew, 126–27
Italian seasoning blend, 206

jalapeño peppers
    Jalapeño-Cilantro Hummus, 62–63
    Jalapeño Cornbread, 37, 45–46
    Mango, Jalapeño & Quinoa Salad,
        91–92
jam (peanut butter substitute), 221
jasmine rice substitute (long-grain
    white rice), 172

Kale
    Kale Apple Dijon Salad, 87–88
kitchen basics
    bakeware, 9, 10
    Budget Byting Principles, 4, 5, 7–9
    chilling food before freezing,
        12–13
    dividing food before freezing, 12
    dry goods, pantry staples, 11
    equipment, 9–11
    freezing food, 5, 8, 12–15
    How to Stock a Kitchen, 5,
        9–11
    ingredients, using wisely, 5, 6, 7–8
    labeling food before freezing, 13
    leftovers, 8
    limitations, freezing food, 13–14
    non-freezer-friendly foods, 13, 15
    packaging for freezing food, 13
    pantry staples, 11–12
    planning meals, 2, 7
    portion control, 9, 12
    pots and pans, 9, 10
    refreezing thawed foods, 14
    refrigerated items, staples, 12
    shopping around, 8–9
    thawing frozen foods, 14
    time ranges for frozen foods, 13–14
    tools, 9, 10–11
    using frozen food, 14
    utensils, 10
    See also Budget Bytes
kneading dough, 38, 40

labeling food before freezing, 13
Lasagna, One-Skillet, 111
learning from failures, 6
leftovers, 8

lemon
    Greek Lemon & Orzo Soup, 138
    Lemon-Butter Green Beans, 204
    Lemon-Garlic Shrimp Pasta,
        175–76
    Lemon-Parmesan Pasta with
        Peas, 115
    Lemon-Raspberry Yogurt Cake,
        216–17
lentils
    Autumn Lentil Pilaf, 186–87
    Lentil & Feta Salad, 83–84
    Lentil & Sausage Stew, 126–27
    tips, 84, 127, 187
    See also beans; rice, beans & lentils
letting dough rise (proofing), 39, 40
Lettuce Wraps, Asian Pork, 171–72
Lighter Ranch Dressing, 72, 207
lime
    Cilantro-Lime Rice, 182
    Creamy Cilantro-Lime Dressing,
        71, 85, 150
    Cumin, Lime & Chickpea Salad,
        71, 85
    Cumin-Lime Sweet Potato Sticks,
        71, 198
    tips, 71, 85, 113
limitations, freezing food, 13–14
linguine (pad thai substitute), 113
Loaded Enchilada Pasta, 77, 104–5
lo mein noodles substitute (fettuccine
    noodles), 153
long-grain white rice (jasmine rice
    substitute), 172

Mac 'n' Chili-Cheese Beef, 146–47
Mango, Jalapeño & Quinoa Salad,
    91–92
mangoes substitute (pineapple), 92
marinade tip, 161
Mashed Potatoes, Triple-Herb,
    211–12
Mason jars for parfaits, 22
mayonnaise
    Teriyaki Salmon with Sriracha
        Mayo, 114, 173–74, 181
    tips, 68, 73
measuring ingredients, 6
meat, poultry & seafood, 141–78
    Asian Pork Lettuce Wraps, 171–72
    Beef & Bean Taquitos, 71, 150–51
    Chicken Tamale Pie, 158–59
    Chili-Cheese Beef 'n' Mac, 146–47
    Chorizo–Sweet Potato Enchiladas,
        164–65
    Coconut Chicken Curry, 154–55

Easy Meat Sauce, 76, 205
Farmer Joes, 142–43
Five-Spice Chops, 166, 181
Ginger Beef 'n' Broccoli, 144–45
Greek Steak Tacos, 148–49
Ham & Swiss Crustless Quiche,
    27–28
Herb-Roasted Pork Loin, 167–68
Lemon-Garlic Shrimp Pasta,
    175–76
Lentil & Sausage Stew, 126–27
Pasta with Tuna & Olives, 109–10
Pork with Balsamic-Cranberry
    Sauce, 169–70
roasting meat, 160
Rosemary-Garlic Roasted Chicken
    & Potatoes, 160–61
slicing meat, 170
Spicy Beef 'n' Noodles, 152–53
Teriyaki Chicken Sliders, 90,
    162–63
Teriyaki Salmon with Sriracha
    Mayo, 114, 173–74, 181
Thai Steamed Fish, 177–78
Turkey Florentine Meatballs,
    156–57
White Beans with Spinach &
    Bacon, 188–89
See also Budget Bytes; chicken
Meatballs, Turkey Florentine, 156–57
meat thermometers, 168
Melon Summer Salad, 82
menus, 5–6, 231–34
metal equipment, 9
Mexican chorizo vs. Spanish
    chorizo, 165
Microwave Apple Crumble for
    One, 218
microwave for thawing frozen
    foods, 14
Mom's Chili (Better-Than), 134–35
Monkey Bread, 226–27
muffins
    Banana-Nut Muffins, 31–32
    Corn Muffins, 45–46
Mug Cake (Chocolate),
    "The One," 221
Multigrain Rolls, 37, 54–55, 132

Naan, 37, 56–57, 124
Newbies Tips, 6
No-Knead Focaccia, 37, 48–49
non-freezer-friendly foods, 13, 15
noodles
    Chinese Chicken Noodle Soup,
        120–21

Spicy Beef 'n' Noodles, 152–53
    See also pasta
Nutella (peanut butter
    substitute), 221
nuts
    Apricot-Walnut Bars, 219
    Banana-Nut Muffins, 31–32
    Chai-Spiced Almonds, 230
    Cranberry-Almond Granola, 24–25

oatmeal
    Autumn Delight Baked Oatmeal,
        20–21
    Banana Bread Baked Oatmeal,
        18–19
oats, old-fashioned rolled oats vs.
    quick-cooking oats, 19
Olives & Tuna, Pasta with, 109–10
"One, The" Chocolate Mug Cake,
    221
One-Skillet Lasagna, 111
Orange-Cranberry Scones, Iced,
    33–34
orange lentils, 84, 127
orzo
    Creamy Orzo with Spinach, 106–7
    Greek Lemon & Orzo Soup, 138

packaging for freezing food, 13
Pad Thai, Easy, 112–13
pantry staples, 11–12
Parfaits, Breakfast, 22–23
Parmesan cheese
    Lemon-Parmesan Pasta with
        Peas, 115
    Parmesan-Herb Drop Biscuits,
        37, 43–44
Parsley & Green Onion Hummus,
    62–63
pasta, 99–117
    Chili-Cheese Beef 'n' Mac, 146–47
    Chinese Chicken Noodle Soup,
        120–21
    Creamy Orzo with Spinach, 106–7
    Easy Pad Thai, 112–13
    freezing pasta tip, 117
    Garlic-Herb Pasta, 108
    Lemon-Garlic Shrimp Pasta,
        175–76
    Lemon-Parmesan Pasta with Peas,
        115
    Loaded Enchilada Pasta, 77, 104–5
    One-Skillet Lasagna, 111
    Pasta e Fagioli, 128–29
    Pasta with Tuna & Olives, 109–10
    Roasted Eggplant Pasta, 102–3

Sesame Noodles, 114
    Spicy Beef 'n' Noodles, 152–53
    Spinach & Artichoke Pasta,
        100–101
    Zucchini-Pasta Bake, 116–17
    See also Budget Bytes
Peach Bubble Cake, 222–23
peanut butter substitute (Nutella,
    jam, caramel sauce), 221
pearled barley, 137
peas
    Curried Potato & Pea Soup,
        130–31
    Lemon-Parmesan Pasta with
        Peas, 115
pies
    Apple Pie Bites, 224–25
    Chicken Tamale Pie, 158–59
Pilaf, Autumn Lentil, 186–87
pineapple
    juice (leftover) tips, 23, 195
    mangoes substitute, 92
    Pineapple Fried Rice, 183
planning meals, 2, 7
    See also Budget Bytes
plastic equipment, 9
poblano peppers tip, 165
pork
    Asian Pork Lettuce Wraps,
        171–72
    Five-Spice Chops, 166, 181
    Herb-Roasted Pork Loin,
        167–68
    menus, 232–33
    pork loin vs. pork tenderloin, 168
    Pork with Balsamic-Cranberry
        Sauce, 169–70
portion control, 9, 12
potatoes
    Curried Potato & Pea Soup,
        130–31
    Dijon Potato & Green Bean Salad,
        94–95
    Indian Skillet Potatoes, 203
    Rosemary-Garlic Roasted
        Chicken & Potatoes, 160–61
    Triple-Herb Mashed Potatoes,
        211–12
pots and pans, kitchen basics,
    9, 10
poultry. See chicken; turkey
preheating your oven, 6
produce markets, 8–9
proofing (letting dough rise),
    39, 40
pumpkin puree, 21

quesadillas
  Chipotle–Sweet Potato Quesadillas,
    208–9
  Strawberry–Cream Cheese
    Quesadillas, 220
Quiche (Crustless), Ham & Swiss,
  27–28
quick breads, 37, 38
Quick Chipotle Black Beans, 184
quick-cooking oats vs. old-fashioned
  rolled oats, 19
Quick Salsa, 64–65
Quinoa, Mango & Jalapeño, 91–92

ramen noodles tip, 121
Ranch Dressing, Lighter, 72, 207
rapid-rise yeast, 39
Raspberry-Lemon Yogurt Cake,
  216–17
reading recipes before beginning, 6
"Real Deal" Chip Dip, The, 68, 207
Red Enchilada Sauce, 77, 104, 105
red lentils, 84, 127, 187
Red Pepper (Roasted) Hummus,
  62–63
red sauce, Easy Meat Sauce, 76, 205
refreezing thawed foods, 14
refrigerated bread/biscuit dough, 227
refrigerated items, staples, 12
refrigerated salads, 88
refrigerator for thawing frozen
  foods, 14
rice, beans & lentils, 179–95
  Autumn Lentil Pilaf, 186–87
  Calico Beans, 193–94
  Cilantro-Lime Rice, 182
  Emerald Rice Salad, 195
  Lentil & Feta Salad, 83–84
  Lentil & Sausage Stew, 126–27
  Pineapple Fried Rice, 183
  Quick Chipotle Black Beans, 184
  rice tip, 172
  Savory Coconut Rice, 181
  Southwest Veggie & Rice Casserole,
    180, 190–91
  Spiced Chickpeas, 185
  Taco Rice, 180, 190
  Tuscan White Beans, 192
  White Beans with Spinach &
    Bacon, 188–89
  See also beans; Budget Bytes
rice cooker, 181
rice vinegar tip, 75
roasting
  Herb-Roasted Pork Loin, 167–68
  meat and, 160

Roasted Broccoli with Crispy
  Garlic, 199–200
Roasted Carrots & Zucchini, 213
Roasted Eggplant Pasta, 102–3
Roasted Red Pepper Hummus,
  62–63
Rosemary-Garlic Roasted Chicken
  & Potatoes, 160–61
Spicy Roasted Eggplant, 201–2
vegetables and, 160, 199
rolled oats (old-fashioned) vs.
  quick-cooking oats, 19
rolls
  Multigrain Rolls, 37, 54–55, 132
  Soft 'n' Sweet Dinner Rolls, 37,
    52–53
  tip, 55
"rooster sauce" (sriracha mayo), 174
Rosemary-Garlic Roasted Chicken &
  Potatoes, 160–61
running water for thawing foods, 14

salads, 79–97
  Apple Dijon Kale Salad, 87–88
  Cumin, Lime & Chickpea Salad,
    71, 85
  customizing, 90
  Dijon Potato & Green Bean Salad,
    94–95
  Easy Asian Slaw, 90
  Emerald Rice Salad, 195
  Greek Chopped Salad, 93
  Lentil & Feta Salad, 83–84
  Mango, Jalapeño & Quinoa Salad,
    91–92
  Southwest Chicken Salad,
    96–97
  Summer Melon Salad, 82
  Super-Crunch Salad, 80–81
  Tomato & White Bean Salad, 89
  Vinaigrette Slaw with Feta, 86
  See also Budget Bytes
Salmon (Teriyaki) with Sriracha
  Mayo, 114, 173–74, 181
Salsa, Quick, 64–65
sambal (chili garlic sauce), 202
sample menus, 5–6, 231–34
sandwiches
  Honey-Wheat Sandwich Bread,
    37, 50–51
  See also dressings, dips & sauces
sauces. See dressings, dips & sauces
Sausage & Lentil Stew, 126–27
Savory Coconut Rice, 181
Scones, Iced Orange-Cranberry,
  33–34

seafood
  Lemon-Garlic Shrimp Pasta,
    175–76
  menus, 233
  Pasta with Tuna & Olives, 109–10
  Teriyaki Salmon with Sriracha
    Mayo, 114, 173–74, 181
Sensible Splurges recipes ($$$), 4, 5
sesame
  Sesame-Ginger Dressing, 74–75
  Sesame Noodles, 114
shopping around, kitchen basics, 8–9
shredded cheese tip, 117
Shrimp (Lemon-Garlic) Pasta, 175–76
skillet dishes
  Chili-Cheese Beef 'n' Mac, 146–47
  Indian Skillet Potatoes, 203
  One-Skillet Lasagna, 111
slaw
  Easy Asian Slaw, 90
  Vinaigrette Slaw with Feta, 86
slicing meat, 170
Sliders, Teriyaki Chicken, 90, 162–63
smoothies, 23, 81, 195
Snow Peas, Ginger, 210
Soft 'n' Sweet Dinner Rolls, 37, 52–53
soups, 119–40
  Better-Than-Mom's Chili, 134–35
  blending hot soups tip, 140
  Broccoli & Cheddar Soup, 132–33
  Carrot–Sweet Potato Soup, 124–25
  Chinese Chicken Noodle Soup,
    120–21
  Curried Potato & Pea Soup,
    130–31
  extra smooth tip, 123
  freezing soups tip, 119
  Greek Lemon & Orzo Soup, 138
  Hearty Vegetable & Barley Soup,
    136–37
  Lentil & Sausage Stew, 126–27
  Pasta e Fagioli, 128–29
  Tomato-Cheddar Soup, 122–23
  Zesty Black Bean Soup, 139–40
  See also Budget Bytes
sour cream substitute (Greek
  yogurt), 68
Southwest-inspired dishes
  Southwest Chicken Salad,
    96–97
  Southwest Veggie & Rice Casserole,
    180, 190–91
Spaghetti Squash, Italian, 205–6
Spiced Chickpeas, 185
spices tip, 155
Spicy Beef 'n' Noodles, 152–53

Spicy Roasted Eggplant, 201–2
spinach
    Creamy Orzo with Spinach, 106–7
    Spinach & Artichoke Pasta,
        100–101
    tips, 81, 107, 189
    Turkey Florentine Meatballs,
        156–57
    White Beans with Spinach &
        Bacon, 188–89
spreads. *See* dressings, dips & sauces
Sriracha Mayo, Teriyaki Salmon with,
    114, 173–74, 181
sriracha mayo ("rooster sauce"), 174
Steak Tacos, Greek, 148–49
Steamed Fish, Thai, 177–78
Stew, Lentil & Sausage, 126–27
stocking a kitchen, 5, 9–11
Strawberry–Cream Cheese
    Quesadillas, 220
sugar (coarse) as icing substitute, 34
Summer Melon Salad, 82
Super-Crunch Salad, 80–81
sweet potatoes
    Carrot–Sweet Potato Soup, 124–25
    Chipotle–Sweet Potato Quesadillas,
        208–9
    Chorizo–Sweet Potato Enchiladas,
        164–65
    Cumin-Lime Sweet Potato Sticks,
        71, 198
    tip, 209
Swiss & Ham Crustless Quiche, 27–28

tacos
    Greek Steak Tacos, 148–49
    Taco Rice, 180, 190
tahini tips, 63, 75
Tamale Pie, Chicken, 158–59
Taquitos, Beef & Bean, 71, 150–51
teriyaki
    Teriyaki Chicken Sliders, 90,
        162–63
    Teriyaki Salmon with Sriracha
        Mayo, 114, 173–74, 181
Thai Steamed Fish, 177–78
thawing frozen foods, 14
thyme tip, 95
time ranges for frozen foods, 13–14
toast
    Apple-Cinnamon French Toast
        Casserole, 35–36
    Avocado-Egg Toast, 30
toasted sesame oil, 75
tomatoes
    Balsamic Tomato Bruschetta, 69–70

tips, 66, 89, 110, 191
Tomato-Cheddar Soup, 122–23
Tomato & White Bean Salad, 89
tomato paste, 194
tools, kitchen basics, 9, 10–11
Triple-Herb Mashed Potatoes, 211–12
Tuna & Olives, Pasta with, 109–10
Turkey Florentine Meatballs, 156–57
Tuscan White Beans, 192

usda.gov, 14
using frozen food, 14
utensils, kitchen basics, 10

vanilla extract tip, 221
vegan recipes
    Apricot-Walnut Bars, 219
    Autumn Lentil Pilaf, 186–87
    Balsamic Tomato Bruschetta, 69–70
    Basic Hummus, 62–63
    Best Bean Dip, 66–67
    Cranberry-Almond Granola, 24–25
    Cumin, Lime & Chickpea Salad,
        71, 85
    Cumin-Lime Sweet Potato Sticks,
        71, 198
    Easy Asian Slaw, 90
    Emerald Rice Salad, 195
    Firecracker Cauliflower,
        72, 207
    Ginger Snow Peas, 210
    Hearty Vegetable & Barley Soup,
        136–37
    Indian Skillet Potatoes, 203
    Italian Breadsticks, 37, 58–59
    Mango, Jalapeño & Quinoa Salad,
        91–92
    Multigrain Rolls, 37, 54–55, 132
    No-Knead Focaccia, 37, 48–49
    Quick Chipotle Black Beans, 184
    Quick Salsa, 64–65
    Red Enchilada Sauce, 77, 104, 105
    Roasted Broccoli with Crispy
        Garlic, 199–200
    Roasted Carrots & Zucchini, 213
    Savory Coconut Rice, 181
    Spiced Chickpeas, 185
    Summer Melon Salad, 82
    Super-Crunch Salad, 80–81
    Taco Rice, 180, 190
    Tomato & White Bean Salad, 89
    Tuscan White Beans, 192
    See also Budget Bytes
vegetable broth (chicken broth
    substitute), 123, 125, 212
vegetables, 197–213

Chipotle–Sweet Potato Quesadillas,
    208–9
Cumin-Lime Sweet Potato Sticks,
    71, 198
Firecracker Cauliflower, 72, 207
frozen vegetables, 197
Ginger Snow Peas, 210
Hearty Vegetable & Barley Soup,
    136–37
Indian Skillet Potatoes, 203
Italian Spaghetti Squash, 205–6
juice tip, 135
Lemon-Butter Green Beans, 204
Roasted Broccoli with Crispy
    Garlic, 199–200
Roasted Carrots & Zucchini, 213
roasting, 160, 199
Southwest Veggie & Rice Casserole,
    180, 190–91
Spicy Roasted Eggplant, 201–2
Triple-Herb Mashed Potatoes,
    211–12
using extra, 121
See also Budget Bytes; dressings,
    dips & sauces; salads; *specific
    vegetables*
vegetarian menus, 234
vegetarian recipes
    Apple-Cinnamon French Toast
        Casserole, 35–36
    Apple Pie Bites, 224–25
    Autumn Delight Baked Oatmeal,
        20–21
    Avocado-Egg Toast, 30
    Banana Bread Baked Oatmeal,
        18–19
    Banana-Nut Muffins, 31–32
    Breakfast Parfaits, 22–23
    Chai-Spiced Almonds, 230
    Cheddar-Beer Bread, 37, 47
    Chipotle–Sweet Potato Quesadillas,
        208–9
    Chocolate-Cherry Biscotti, 228–29
    Creamy Balsamic Dressing, 73, 80
    Creamy Cilantro-Lime Dressing,
        71, 85, 150
    Creamy Orzo with Spinach, 106–7
    Dijon Potato & Green Bean Salad,
        94–95
    Easy Pad Thai, 112–13
    Garlic-Herb Pasta, 108
    Greek Chopped Salad, 93
    Honey-Wheat Biscuits, 37, 41–42
    Honey-Wheat Sandwich Bread,
        37, 50–51
    Huevos Rancheros Bowls, 29

vegetarian recipes (*cont.*)
  Iced Orange-Cranberry Scones, 33–34
  Italian Baked Eggs, 26
  Italian Spaghetti Squash, 205–6
  Jalapeño Cornbread, 37, 45–46
  Lemon-Butter Green Beans, 204
  Lemon-Parmesan Pasta with Peas, 115
  Lemon-Raspberry Yogurt Cake, 216–17
  Lentil & Feta Salad, 83–84
  Lighter Ranch Dressing, 72, 207
  Microwave Apple Crumble for One, 218
  Monkey Bread, 226–27
  Naan, 37, 56–57, 124
  "One, The" Chocolate Mug Cake, 221
  Parmesan-Herb Drop Biscuits, 37, 43–44
  Peach Bubble Cake, 222–23
  "Real Deal" Chip Dip, The, 68, 207
  Roasted Eggplant Pasta, 102–3

Sesame-Ginger Dressing, 74–75
Sesame Noodles, 114
Soft 'n' Sweet Dinner Rolls, 37, 52–53
Southwest Veggie & Rice Casserole, 180, 190–91
Spinach & Artichoke Pasta, 100–101
Strawberry–Cream Cheese Quesadillas, 220
Vinaigrette Slaw with Feta, 86
Zucchini-Pasta Bake, 116–17
See also Budget Bytes
Vinaigrette Slaw with Feta, 86
volume conversions, 238

Walnuts
  Apple Dijon Kale Salad, 87–88
  Apricot-Walnut Bars, 219
  Autumn Delight Baked Oatmeal, 20–21
  Banana Bread Baked Oatmeal, 18–19
  Banana-Nut Muffins, 31–32

wheat
  Honey-Wheat Biscuits, 37, 41–42
  Honey-Wheat Sandwich Bread, 37, 50–51
white beans
  Tomato & White Bean Salad, 89
  Tuscan White Beans, 192
  White Beans with Spinach & Bacon, 188–89
white wine substitute (chicken broth), 101
wood equipment, 9
Wraps (Lettuce), Asian Pork, 171–72

yeast breads, 37, 38–40
yeasts, 38–39, 49
yellow lentils, 84, 127, 187
Yogurt Cake, Lemon-Raspberry, 216–17
yogurt tip, 217

Zesty Black Bean Soup, 139–40
zucchini
  Roasted Carrots & Zucchini, 213
  Zucchini-Pasta Bake, 116–17